# PRAISE FOR
## VACCINES & BAYONETS

"At a time when vaccines are front page news and a deadly pandemic is raging across the globe, Bee Bloeser's memoir of her family's role in US smallpox eradication efforts in Africa during the late 1960s makes for riveting reading. Set against the backdrop of civil war in Nigeria and a brutal postcolonial dictatorship in Equatorial Guinea, Bloeser's book is both a captivating family history and a reminder—fifty years later—of how public health campaigns are still inextricably intertwined with politics. Today, as superpowers trade blame for the spread of a deadly disease and wealthy nations hoard lifesaving vaccine supplies while the rest vie for what remains, *Vaccines and Bayonets* illustrates how inoculating vulnerable people against a killer virus can be a tool of soft power that builds diplomatic goodwill in the darkest of times and offers a glimpse of what the US government is capable of achieving when it chooses to lead, rather than retreat, in the face of a global pandemic."

—Sasha Polakow-Suransky,
Deputy Editor of *Foreign Policy* magazine and author of
*Go Back to Where You Came From: The Backlash Against Immigration and the Fate of Western Democracy*

"Bee Bloeser has written a closely observed and revealing memoir of her family's experience living first in northern Nigeria and then in the tropical island capital of Equatorial Guinea half a century ago. In both of the newly independent countries they joined a successful fight against smallpox. They also relished the opportunity of living in richly different and stimulating cultures. With affectionate detail she relates how her husband, Carl, and his teams of local vaccinators contributed to a global effort to eradicate a disease that had maimed and killed on a terrifying scale. That experience was historically important, not least in the light of new, urgent, global efforts to deliver vaccinations to defeat the coronavirus pandemic. This account is most remarkable when it relates the family's experiences as Americans living in tropical, isolated and unfortunate Equatorial Guinea, a tiny country then enduring the "terror"—the violent rule of a capricious dictator, Macias Nguema. Although their [official] status offered some protection, the young family faced the threat of detention while their local friends and colleagues faced the threat of torture or worse at the hands of the authorities. Equatorial Guinea has gone on, ever since, to suffer more decades of violence, attempted coup-plots and much wider misfortune. Bee Bloeser's memoir is a reminder that misrule and fear blighted the country from the start of its modern existence. This is a sympathetic, vividly told and useful record of an unusually sombre moment in West African history."

—Adam Roberts,

*The Economist* Midwest Correspondent, previously in Paris, Bureau Chief in Delhi and Johannesburg; author of *The Wonga Coup* and *Superfast Primetime Ultimate Nation*

"Bloeser's story reads like a political thriller, women's history, and African adventure rolled into one. An alert witness to a breakthrough in world health, she brings insight and humor to a dark tale of disease, corruption and genocide that unfolds around her, her visionary but practical husband, and their two small children. Naïve, she scrambles to adjust to life in Africa—then finds herself falling with her young children into a terrifying political nightmare that continues even after she returns to the U.S. Riveting."

—Pamela Alexander,
Pulitzer Prize-nominated author,
Creative writing faculty, MIT and Oberlin College

"Bee Bloeser's engrossing memoir is a loving and beautifully written testament to the hard work, determination and considerable self-sacrifice required to eliminate a disfiguring, deadly disease from the earth. It takes perseverance, guts, and a heart for humanity to do what these public health workers and their families achieved, and live to tell about it. The world owes them a debt of gratitude."

—Andrea Arthur Owan, M.S., A.T., R.,
Public Health Professional, Published Author, Speaker
and IFOC Senior Chaplain-Ordained

"I just finished reading *Vaccines & Bayonets*. I am simply blown away by your detailed writing, your ability to tell this gripping story, the life experiences you had in Africa and the courageous woman you were and are to live there and reach back to tell this story."

—Ethel Lee-Miller,
Enhanced Life Management-Author,
Public Speaker, Writing Seminar

"Bee Bloeser will engage and move you deeply while sharing her personal journey in Africa during the eradication of smallpox. With a backdrop of corruption, genocide, and oppression of women, she still provides an insightful tapestry of victories won and hope for the future. Highly recommend."

—Linda Herzog, J.D.

"Evocative and powerful. When does a historical memoir forewarn us of major events repeating this moment in today's headlines? Bloeser rides as wife and clear-eyed witness alongside her husband on his vaccination mission. You can't make her stories up, nor will you put this book down."

—Sally A. Raymond, M.A.,
Psychotherapist, Speaker and Author:
*The Son I Knew Too Late:*
*A Guide to Help You Survive and Thrive*

# VACCINES & BAYONETS

FIGHTING SMALLPOX IN AFRICA

AMID TRIBALISM, TERROR AND THE

COLD WAR

A Historical Memoir

## BEE BLOESER

Published by Wheatmark®
2030 East Speedway Boulevard, Suite 106
Tucson, Arizona 85719 USA
www.wheatmark.com

BIOGRAPHY & AUTOBIOGRAPHY / Personal Memoirs
HISTORY / Africa / West
MEDICAL / History

Front cover design by Le Studio Raw.

ISBN: 978-1-62787-856-2 (paperback)
ISBN: 978-1-62787-857-9 (hardcover)
ISBN: 978-1-62787-858-6 (ebook)
LCCN: 2021900782

Bulk ordering discounts are available through Wheatmark, Inc.
For more information, email orders@wheatmark.com
or call 1-888-934-0888.

rev202101

For Carl, who more than anyone I know always tried to do the right thing, who loved deeply, who showed me the world, who departed this life too soon.

And for Charles and Ginger, who lived through interesting times with us in far corners of the world.

[Smallpox eradication] required the right people: doctors, epidemiologists, administrators, and volunteers who risked their safety and sanity in pursuit of an elusive goal . . .

—Bob H. Reinhardt, *The End of a Global Pox: America and the Eradication of Smallpox in the Cold War Era*

# CONTENTS

## Part II
### If You Scream and Nobody Hears . . .

Part III

The Turning Point

Part IV

The Long Shadow

## Epilogue

# PREFACE

*This is a* work of nonfiction—part memoir, part history. The events included are as true as I can remember them over the span of fifty years and as supported by my collection of contemporaneous, unclassified primary documents. Some memories were triggered by input from others who are a part of this history—writings by those now deceased and interviews with the few still living. The people named in *Vaccines & Bayonets* are real and not composites. In some instances, I have compressed multiple encounters into one when doing so did not change the truth of what happened. Information presented in letter form is composed from content of my actual letters or cassette-tape letters, from diary notes in my archives and from added contextual material. Dialogue and gestures are either as I recorded them in letters I wrote at the time or are created to report as accurately as possible the way I remember the interactions. For a more complete discussion, see "On Writing *Vaccines & Bayonets*" at the end of this book.

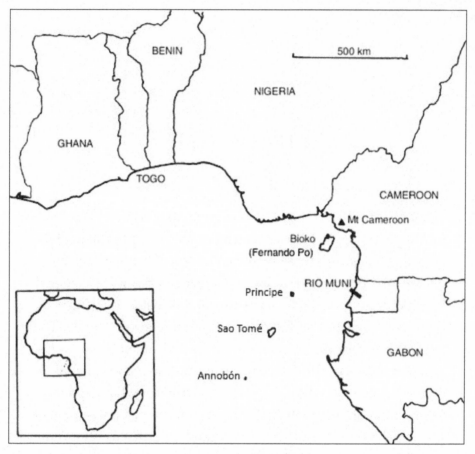

1. Kano is in north central Nigeria, just off the edge of this map.
2. Equatorial Guinea consists of Fernando Po (now Bioko), Rio Muni and Annobón.

# PROLOGUE

*It was called* the Cold War. The powerful eyed the resource-rich continent of Africa with its newly and soon-to-be independent countries. China, Russia and her allies, America and hers all purchased loyalty with aid. They fought proxy wars. They maneuvered to outwit each other in now widely documented espionage. But amid these intrigues and power plays, there was a mutual enemy against which all nations had common cause. A virus and the disease it caused. A disease with no cure and no treatment. Smallpox.

In this Cold War context, my husband, Carl, and I, with two young children and wide-eyed ideals, moved to West Africa in the global war to defeat the virus and consign it to the history books. Carl passionately joined the battle. I eagerly followed him into a world completely foreign to my small-town roots, first to a country that was always in the news and then to one that should have been.

The first: Nigeria. Larger than the US state of Texas. Embroiled in a civil war, the Nigeria-Biafra War. If others hadn't cared about Africans killing Africans, they did care about starving Biafran babies. Images sped around the globe. The powerful chose sides. The world watched and wept.

Our second assignment: Equatorial Guinea. A tiny dot on the globe, smaller than the US state of Maryland. Newly independent and with no reports escaping its borders, it was plunged into a reign of terror. A blanket of fear muffled its screams. The powerful chose silence. The world didn't watch, didn't weep, didn't even know the place existed.

While my husband fought on the frontlines of the battle between human and microbe—and took on "other duties as assigned" in America's smallest embassy—our family was isolated in an isolated country, a frontline of a different sort. I made cryptic notes and hid them in the sock drawer.

Through the ages, disease has shifted the centers of power. Smallpox dethroned dynasties and defeated armies. It killed on average 30 percent of its victims—totaling over 300 million deaths in the twentieth century alone—and left too many survivors blind, deformed and disfigured.

Smallpox was an enemy so dreaded that nations on opposite sides of an ideological divide joined a common battle to send it into history as the first human disease ever eradicated. That global assault succeeded. The disease is gone. The virus isn't. Despite heated debates, samples of the virus are still kept in high-security laboratory freezers—legally, only in one location in the US and one in Russia. Extreme vigilance aims to prevent escape, accidental or otherwise.

Just as disease alters power and politics, world powers use disease *fighters* to do the same. Governments dispense aid with an eye on the influence and goodwill it will purchase—the soft power angle. Leading off in the coordinated global fight to rid the world of smallpox gave America a means to do good *and* pursue those foreign policy interests.

Now, as then, individuals and their families, sent by governments, nongovernmental organizations (NGOs), missions and corporations, may be in harm's way. They are often minute parts of a vast and complex geopolitical strategy and go into isolated and poorly understood situations. They may be required to deftly navigate relations between the home country and a hostile government. They battle diseases like Ebola and SARS, yes, but also terror, oppression of women, child sex trafficking and despotic rulers. Like me, naïve dependents may find themselves facing physical and emotional challenges for which they are ill prepared.

The fact that the war on smallpox served foreign policy interests takes nothing away from the lives saved, the gift of the vaccine or the startling enormity of the globally coordinated victory. In *The End of a Global Pox*, author Bob Reinhardt alludes to smallpox chronicles that recount feats of derring-do that made eradication possible and that tell of the heroes who risked safety and sanity in pursuit of the goal.

As complex as the broader picture may be, this first-person history tells of the Africa and the smallpox campaign I experienced with one of those heroes.

# PART I

# THE CALLING

# 1

# RANKA DIDI

*Meninge urged our* double-cab truck over washboard roads and cow tracks as we pressed north in the direction of the Sahara. In the front seat with his driver, my husband leaned forward, searching the horizon. At the last mud-walled village, he'd learned that a group of nomads was camped nearer Nigeria's border with Niger, and he had to find them before they moved on. With no new case of smallpox reported for several weeks, this was a high-risk period when people might let down their guard. Carl and his teams had to search for and quickly quarantine any new case to prevent reintroduction of the disease.

From the back seat I peered out through the fine dust. Twenty-foot termite hills—spires of ochre clay—anchored a ghostly landscape that dissolved into white sky. An occasional camel grazed on thorn bush and stunted acacia.

We knew exactly what was at stake. More than once today out here in the Sahel, this belt between Sahara and savanna, people had appeared out of nowhere, many with skin covered by the ugly, hard-earned smallpox survivor badge. Running toward our truck, they raised their fists and shouted, *"Ranka didi!"* May you live long! Then the ululation—the long, emotional, high-pitched trilling sound. It was a common response to our white Dodge

3

Power Wagon with its USAID logo and its blue-lettered sign announcing the smallpox eradication program.

Meninge pumped the brakes, and the truck shuddered to a stop. Grateful for whatever had interrupted our bone-jarring ride, I shifted to look out the front window. A few tired stragglers from a herd of the Sahel's white, bony, long-horned dairy cattle had decided to lie down in the road. A Fulani boy of about ten herded his family's wealth. A girl bearing a calabash of milk on her head was a few yards farther on. As we waited for the boy to collect the last of his herd, the acrid smell of dung floated into the cab. Then, through the scrub I saw five or six huts enclosed by a fence of sticks. A handful of people emerged, ran to the road shouting their salutes and closed around our truck.

Among those closest to my window were two women, a mother and daughter perhaps. The older woman's eyes locked with mine, and tears streamed down her cheeks. "Ranka didi!"

Perhaps the younger woman had been beautiful—before smallpox. With her deep, pitted scars, she could manage only a hint of a smile. But her vision had been spared, and it seemed that an urgent light burned in eyes framed by pockmarks where eyelashes should have been. I recoiled inside, fought to keep my face from revealing the wave of nausea and forced myself to look into her eyes. *That's it. Concentrate. Just focus on her eyes.*

I knew about viruses. I knew that when a virus finishes using one cell, one person, one host, leaving it damaged or dead, it has to find a new one so it can continue making copies of itself. And then find another. And another. It's what a virus has to do. And I knew a lot about smallpox, caused by the *variola* virus. I knew that more than a few times through the ages, the microscopic organism had changed the course of history itself. I knew the disease had come closer than any other to annihilating entire civilizations.

And I knew there was no cure. Not in the Yoruba smallpox god, Shapona, and not in the leaves of the neem tree. Once granted access to the body, nothing could stop the virus. Nothing could slow it down. Yes, I knew many facts that the two women did not.

But they knew the smell of smallpox. Could sense it from yards away. The smell of decaying flesh, like that of a dead animal. The young woman would know its aches, chills, fever and nausea. She knew the stealth of smallpox, for after she seemed to recover from the flu-like symptoms, the virus suddenly leapt from hiding. It planted sores in her mouth and raced across her forehead, then the rest of her face, stealing her beauty, then down her body to the palms of her hands, the soles of her feet. It persisted until it filled the hideous sores with pus, white, then yellow, drawing flies with its putrid odor.

And she knew the aloneness of the isolation hut, and in that dark space knew hunger when sores in her mouth and throat made it too painful to swallow. She knew agony from the unseen lesions on internal organs and from bedding brushed against pustules beginning to break down. And then, after defying the odds and surviving smallpox, she would have known emotional isolation as friends averted their eyes. And worse, the horror in the eyes of her husband when he tried to look at her.

The older woman may have sat outside the restricted hut, cooking a soup in the desperate hope her daughter could swallow a little of it. As she kept vigil, she could have known heartbreaking memories of children she had buried after their gruesome deaths, and now the fear of losing one more.

Yes, these women knew smallpox.

They knew that before the big white trucks came, a third of their family infected with smallpox had died and that many who survived were left disfigured and blinded. And as well as they knew anything, they knew that the virus could have taken the little boy playing at their feet.

The older woman cried as she picked up the toddler, his skin smooth as silk, and proudly held him up to show me.

"Ranka didi! Ranka didi!"

We were engaged in all-out war to annihilate smallpox. The battle had a long history that the women would not know. They didn't know about eighteenth-century inoculations or the decades of development behind the vaccine or the invention of the rapid-fire injector or the contact tracing in a race against time. They didn't know that right across the border in Niger, on November 30, 1969, the campaign had given its 100-millionth vaccination. And they did not know that throughout history, no human disease had ever been eradicated or that countless experts declared we could not eradicate this one.

But these women with tear-stained faces gratefully showing me the child knew the campaign against smallpox in a way that Carl and I never could. They knew that because the big white trucks came, bringing fellow Nigerians with the vaccines, smallpox had been denied access to the body of this handsome little boy, that his cousins had also escaped and that their family was still able to raise the cattle and sell the milk.

As the last few cows surrendered their resting place in the road and ambled into the sparse scrub of the African Sahel, Meninge shifted gears and we were underway. I'd had my first intimate look at smallpox, and I didn't even try to hold back the tears. The two women and their neighbors, arms still held high, watched our truck for a long time, not yet knowing that smallpox had visited their huts for the last time.

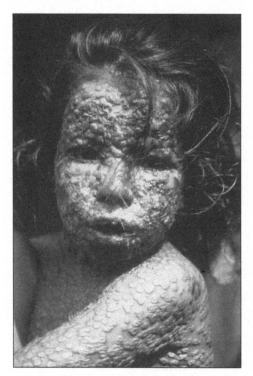

A young smallpox victim

# 2

## CALLED TO AFRICA

*Six Months Earlier*

A lot of Oklahoma girls wanted to go to Dallas. I wanted to go to Africa. I'd always wanted to go to Africa. And here I was—boarding Pan American World Airways as the sun set on JFK International. Carl and I, our four-year-old son, Charles, and eighteen-month-old daughter, Ginger, were taking a step that felt as epic to me as Neil Armstrong's "giant leap for mankind" onto the moon a few weeks before.

In that zone of too excited to sleep and too exhausted to do otherwise, I fantasized that Charles and Ginger would be in dreamland for hours after our already tiring day of multiple plane changes. I pulled pillows and blankets from the bin above our bulkhead seats and optimistically constructed our nest for the seventeen-hour flight to Lagos, Nigeria. Carl rolled his eyes and groaned as the three young men in the next row whooped the opening toast of a transatlantic party.

The stewardesses, as they were called then, all looking like models out of *Vogue*, removed their white gloves and perky hats and served dinner. By the time they gathered the trays and the clinking of china and silver died away, the next row's decibel level began to climb. Between fitful catnaps, wrapped in the economy cabin's coarse blanket and recycled air, my mind touched down here and there on events that had led to this life-altering move.

Born Rubye Lee Harbin (later nicknamed Bee), an Oklahoma minister's daughter, I grew up in a happy, stable family with my parents and younger sister, and with another seven happy, stable families in my large extended one. Everything was ordered and predictable and safe in my world.

I wanted adventure. I was curious about lives far beyond my provincial one, whether Far Beyond was across the ocean or across the tracks. I devoured stories and filmstrips of doctors and nurses working in jungles, especially those from a great uncle and a cousin who served in Africa.

And then there was my theatrical self. Mother and Daddy had enrolled me in what were then called expression lessons, where I recited poetry and monologues. After my five-year-old voice went out over the airwaves of Oklahoma City's WKY radio, I was launched as the family's featured entertainer.

As my theatrical bent married my Africa obsession, I played the lead, living in a jungle hut in the scenes staged in my head. These all shaped my 1947 carefully executed cursive tenth-birthday diary entry titled "What I Want to Be When I Grow Up."

My Africa goal came second, of course, to marrying Mr. Right. Better yet, Mr. Right would take me to Africa, and together we'd have the self-sacrificing adventure that life in the bush was sure to provide.

Fast-forward to a fall evening in 1960. The piece of paper granting me all the rights and privileges pertaining to a bachelor's degree in theater was still warm under my arm when I agreed to a blind date with a guy named Carl Bloeser.

He had just returned from serving three years at the US Air Force hospital in Wiesbaden, Germany, as a surgical nurse and an air evacuation medic. Those specialties had ignited his life's passion.

Carl correctly sensed I was a kindred spirit and didn't wait past the second date to tell me his goal was to work in medical missions. Six months later we were married.

For a long while, Africa remained on the back burner. Our children arrived while I completed a master's degree in speech pathology—a more practical career choice than theater—so I focused on studying, working to help make ends meet and washing diapers.

Carl had challenging work in the US Public Health Service's venereal disease program. He proved to be a natural at epidemiology. After completing his lengthy interview-and-investigation training in New York City, he set records in preventing disease transmission with his contact-tracing success. He worked first in the hills of Arkansas, then in the cities and broad expanses of New Mexico, and finally in Native American pueblos and on the Navajo, Hopi and Zuni reservations.

At the same time, he earned his master's degree in public administration, with a focus on healthcare (he would later complete a master's in public health), so we were too busy and preoccupied to talk about the dream that had drawn us together.

But my husband was a man of mystery, a man I would come to know—and not know—over the years. I had not yet realized a topic could occupy a major place in his thoughts without my knowing it.

On a snowy Santa Fe, New Mexico day in 1969, Carl rushed in the door from work, breathless and grinning like a little kid. It had come—The Call—from the West Africa Smallpox Eradication/Measles Control Program. I had no idea he had applied. A program manager flew from Atlanta, Georgia, to interview Carl and then me. After a long selection process, they concluded our family was a good fit for the program, and Carl signed on as an operations officer. We were moving to Kano, Nigeria! Mr. Right was indeed taking me to Africa!

Fortified with every vaccine I had ever heard of and some I hadn't, we left New Mexico for the life of our dreams. But the first stop was three months in Atlanta, where the new crop of operations officers, medical epidemiologists, and Epidemic Intelligence Service (EIS) officers received intensive training at the National Communicable Disease Center (NCDC). We often shortened it to CDC.

Some announcement from the cockpit brought me back from the fresh air of memory lane to a half-dazed awareness of our confined space. I shifted again in my endless quest for comfort and dozed off and on, mostly off, courtesy of the merrymakers. I thought I might as well review our State Department protocol booklet for Americans on *official* status in a foreign country.

"Representation of the United States of America." Oh my goodness. It sounded so important. I pictured myself in poised and perceptive conversations with foreign dignitaries, one of my many illusions of a life of international service. I could not know then the darker meaning the word "representation" would acquire for our family just a year in the future.

Across the aisle, Carl was annoyingly sound asleep. Probably dreaming of the challenge ahead. A tough job? Good. Formidable? Better. Nigh impossible? Best. Bring it on.

During training in Atlanta, a few classes for spouses—taught by couples returning from Africa—covered health, safety, household management and culture shock. It might have been helpful to hear from immigrant families. Immigrants have been uprooted, they've dealt with it, they've managed. They could have given insight into how a couple, and young children, adjust to life in a turbulent time. But then, I wasn't anticipating a turbulent time.

I took the children around Atlanta for experiences that would be unavailable for the next two years—museums, a fire station, an auto assembly plant, and a live children's television show. We dined with fellow trainees and formed friendships.

At one evening get-together, I overheard a colleague comment that he would never accept an assignment to Equatorial Guinea, given all the trouble going on there. I'd never heard of the place. The country wasn't in the smallpox eradication program, so I didn't know why he made the comment. He probably went on to tell some details, but I was talking with his wife. I wasn't listening.

Everyone was lined up and stuck with more needles. More entries on that yellow immunization card. I don't remember which made everyone's children scream the loudest—typhoid, typhus or the three-shot rabies series. Our official US passports were stamped with Nigerian visas, official passports providing more privileges and protections than a regular one, but not as many as a diplomatic passport.

At the end of training, and after Carl's two-week detail to the Gulf Coast to assist in the public health crisis created by Hurricane Camille, the day arrived. We were on our way to Nigeria, suitcases and spirits bursting at the seams.

I looked down at Charles, his head resting on my arm, my reading light highlighting his blond hair and his souvenirs of our flight—pilot's wings and a little Pan Am plane. Charles was always a good sleeper, a blessing through our late-night study sessions in grad school.

Ginger had her dad's olive complexion and dark hair but, sadly, not his ability to sleep through a lot of noise. As time zones came and went, the young men in the row behind us had more rounds of drinks. Each time their party gathered new steam, Ginger cried with renewed vigor. My husband still slept.

This man of mine could be a puzzle. Enigmatic. That was the

word. It was like there was a part of his life I would never be privy to. *I wonder what he's dreaming.*

Flying into the first tint of dawn somewhere past the mid Atlantic, I mentally searched the unseen path ahead. Despite extensive orientation in Atlanta, a great unknown stretched before us once our feet touched African soil. My memory sifted through the images that had formed childhood dreams—and I couldn't wait.

I reached across the aisle for Carl's hand. He'd been oblivious to the crying and partying. How was it possible? Waking up now, he pushed his bolo tie up closer to his rumpled shirt collar and stroked the dark stubble of a beard he'd started growing during hurricane fieldwork. Maybe he wanted to make up for the thinning hair on top. I hadn't yet decided whether I liked it.

*Look at that smile. He can't wait either.* He had previous international experience from his years in the air force, and in public health he had slogged through a quagmire of tragedies as he worked reservations and inner-city streets. So his perspective would be practical and more realistic than mine.

At least a dozen hours into the flight, during approach into Dakar, I scooted over to the window seat, a frenzied tap dance going on in my chest as I got my first glimpse of the continent. Africa! I could hardly believe it.

On the ground for maybe a half hour, we weren't allowed to deplane. But we were near the open door, and I got a whiff of Africa's enticing smells and heard her unfamiliar sounds. Approaching Monrovia and Accra, our other stops along the coast, and finally Lagos, as our descent brought us low enough to see detail on the ground, I pressed my forehead against the pane. Below us, dense jungle often opened its dark green canopy to reveal a cluster of thatch-roofed huts. Children ran out to wave. Misty columns of gray pinpointed cooking fires. The canopy always closed as abruptly as it opened, but an occasional meandering line of silver forced it open again, a river that looked clean and clear from the air.

I couldn't foresee the atrocities that would soon invade my naïve view of Africa or the effects of physical and emotional isolation I would experience. Or the grim way in which man's inhumanity to man would exhibit itself within our own ranks.

My mind gripped the *National Geographic*–like image it had created. I saw the Africa I imagined. No disturbing realities yet marred the vision.

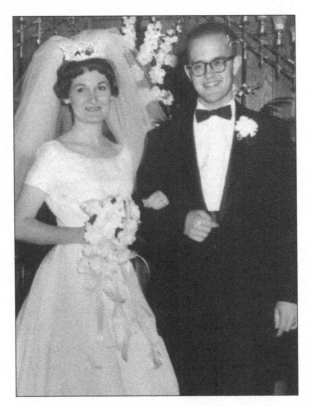

Bee and Carl on their wedding day, 1961

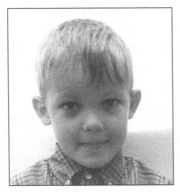 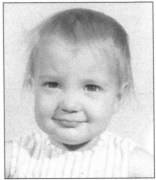

Charles and Ginger, passport photos, 1969

# 3

# TO THE SAHEL

*Landing in Lagos,* someone had told us, simulated stepping into warm Saran Wrap. I agreed when we stepped out of the plane into the steamy arms of sweet, heavy air.

Despite the toll of the seventeen-hour flight, every unfamiliar sound, smell and sight on the long ride from the airport was a shot of adrenaline. I thought I'd be deafened by the symphony of bells, horns, shouts and music and get dizzy trying to look in all directions at once. The color! To my Western eye, women's three wardrobe components—cotton wrapper (the two-meter length of fabric wrapped around the lower body like a skirt), blouse, and turban—seemed to have been chosen to clash with each other in every way color and pattern could clash. An arresting sensory riot.

I kept pinching myself. *I-am-in-Africa!*

With sheer bravado, drivers of cars, lorries, bicycles and motor scooters forged their way through the mass of humanity, and the American smallpox operations officer taking us to our hotel had learned to hold his own. I was too mesmerized to be frightened.

We would be in Lagos for an orientation week before proceeding on to Kano. Dr. Stan Foster, head of the Smallpox Measles Program (SMP) for Nigeria, and his family offered the ultimate in kind hospitality. Charles played with the Foster boys. The African women took turns giving Ginger rides in slings on their backs. Mrs. Foster showed me African household challenges and clever ways over, around or through them.

Carl spent the days with Stan and the program operations people. This coordinated regional war on smallpox covered nineteen (eventually twenty) contiguous countries in West and Central Africa. If zero pox was achieved here, global eradication could be considered a realistic goal. The US Agency for International Development (USAID) funded and CDC led the charge. And now that the United States was enthusiastically onboard, the World Health Organization (WHO) began to staff its stalled global campaign.

The countries in this part of Africa were desperate for some control of measles, a devastating child killer in the region, and insisted we also address that problem. Hence, the West and Central Africa Smallpox Eradication-Measles Control Program (SMP). Informally, we found various paths to brevity—often just smallpox-measles program, and sometimes in casual conversation, simply smallpox program or SMP. WHO's global campaign was the Smallpox Eradication Program (SEP).

In the evening, the Fosters regaled us with smallpox program stories. My favorite involved Dr. Bill Foege, our beloved chief of operations. His name was spoken with equal parts awe and affection around here, as it had been in Atlanta. At six-foot-seven, Bill stood out in any crowd. One day when working in eastern Nigeria, he told the chief of a large village he could protect the entire village population against smallpox if the chief would get everyone to a vaccination assembly point. The chief didn't need to set up a committee to study the proposal. He immediately turned and said something to his village messenger, who set to work on the talking drum. People streamed into the village market, and with the jet injector, Bill vaccinated several thousand in a few hours. At the end of the day, he asked the chief what message he had sent that got the people to drop everything in the middle of a workday and come so quickly. The chief had told them to come to the market if they wanted to see the tallest man in the world.

Everyone involved in stamping out the scourge of smallpox had a herculean task ahead. They approached it with absolute confidence that eradication would be achieved. Because the main challenge to that goal was one of management, not medicine, the program had at least twice as many operations officers as it had physician epidemiologists. The physician for our area was posted in Kaduna, so from Lagos we flew up-country to spend a few days with him and his wife before going on to our new home in Kano. They gave us insight into living and working in Nigeria's Muslim north.

Carl sipped his coffee, strong and black, as they educated us about regional hatreds, attacks and counterattacks. One of the major flashpoints, in Kano, had led to the current civil war and the fighting now confined to a small section of eastern Nigeria.

War? I had completely forgotten about the Nigeria-Biafra war. Where were the signs of it? There'd been a few soldiers at the Lagos airport, and I think we saw one barricaded building in the city. Other than that, we'd seen no indication of a country in the grip of a civil war, and I'd heard no conversation about it. I didn't know it then, but on the CBS show *60 Minutes*, filmed in Nigeria at the time, Harry Reasoner talked about the "staggering normalcy" in all but 10 percent of the country. That 10 percent was eight hundred miles away.

Saying goodbye to our hosts, we flew to our final destination in Kano. Carl was ready to take the reins of his program. From the little Nigerian Airways Fokker Friendship, I looked down at a horizon-to-horizon carpet of brown, actually beige—the parched Sahel, that transition belt between Sahara and savannah. I squeezed Carl's hand as the pilot set the plane down and we taxied into our future.

—➤

A rush of hot air and a friendly "Mr. Bloeser, welcome to Kano" greeted us as we stepped onto the tarmac.

Carl looked up into the face of a slender, white-robed African man. With his reserved smile, Meninge, the program's driver-interpreter, said something like, "Sir, it is good that you arrive safe. Now I will take you to your house. You rest, sir. Tomorrow I will come for you and take you to your office." His British English melded with rhythms of his native dialect.

Meninge loaded our luggage into the SMP's freshly scrubbed white Dodge Power Wagon while Carl helped the kids and me into the back seat.

Carl needed to get to know this man with whom he would spend long days, both in the city and in the bush. He asked questions, and Meninge gave short answers. Not abrupt, but brief. He was Yoruba, he said, from western Nigeria, Yoruba Land. But he had lived up here among the Hausa and Fulani for several years, was fluent in the language and was Muslim.

Crowds cheered us and ululated as we passed them in our smallpox program Power Wagon. I felt a rush of pride. A thrill. We would be making history.

Mud buildings, primarily one story, made the city look like a bunch of little matchboxes crowded against each other. Billboards, splashes of color against the beige, promoted infant formula, shoes, beer and anti-malaria pills.

An occasional three- or four-story building and escalating

traffic signaled our approach to the city center. Motorized traffic here, less chaotic than the free-for-all in Lagos, where honking horns set the rules of the road, was often slowed by lumbering, two-wheeled wooden carts. Massive loads topped the flatbed conveyances, and six or seven muscular men, their torsos bent close to horizontal with the effort, provided the power.

The *mammy wagon*, more lorry than bus, was the ubiquitous mass transit vehicle. Wide-spaced horizontal wood slats formed the sides of the converted truck, and people, chickens or even a goat bulged through the gaps. Bundles were piled on top. Extra passengers—it seemed every mammy wagon had them—stationed themselves on a running-board, clutching one of the slats. Painted mottos like "The Lord is My Shepherd," "Slow but Sure" or "A Good Friend is Like Gold" graced the sides and front.

I'd never been so excited, so fascinated.

We did pass several beggars. And I had a brief glimpse of men disfigured by smallpox or leprosy. But I still clung to the romanticized picture in my head.

Half an hour from the airport, we drove into a neighborhood where houses sat on wide yards of dust. Pink- and white-blossomed oleander bushes bordered each property. Tires crunched on the gravel as Meninge made a right turn into the driveway of a boxy two-story house. White plaster covered the block construction of the house and the two-room servants' quarters out back. White decorative walls made of alternating cinder blocks and open spaces defined a carport and half the front perimeter.

As we climbed out of the truck, a man of medium height and stocky build bounded out of the house and rushed toward us, wearing an enormous smile.

"Ah! Sir! Welcome to your house. We be waiting for you!" His eagerness and booming voice felt overwhelming.

"Ah, Mister Charles, Miss Ginger. Come. See." Adamu had obviously been briefed on our family names. "Charles, you goin' be Africa man." Ginger gripped my skirt, and Charles dropped behind Carl.

A whiff of bleach stung my nose as Adamu opened the door to our African home. The floor nearly sparkled, so I removed my shoes as Adamu led the way for a tour of the house we were to live in for the next two years. His enthusiasm never waned.

A modest living room/dining room, an adequate kitchen, a toilet and a tiny guest room were on the ground floor. Upstairs, one average-size bedroom, two smaller ones and a full-size bathroom completed the picture. I remember the flooring felt smooth and cool to my feet—some kind of linoleum, I think. The basic furniture looked semicomfortable.

I told Carl I thought the house was nice. And roomy. I'm not sure why I bothered to say that. He never cared about a house, and he hated it when anyone referred to houses as homes. He always said, "Why does anyone need a big house? All you need is shelter—four walls and a roof." His attitude on cars? One only needed to get from point A to point B—an engine, four wheels and a steering wheel. Well, yes, and seats.

Glass louvered windows, both upstairs and down, created an open, bright environment. An obvious scrub-down with bleach or some kind of cleaner and a coat of fresh paint had prepared the house for our arrival. Yes, I liked it. I was fine with its not being the jungle hut of my fantasies.

I was taken aback, though, to learn that Adamu was not there just to get the house ready and to greet us. He and his wife and little girl were installed in the servant quarters behind the house.

I had sworn never to have servants! Did USAID just assume we would hire him? I'd been in Kano thirty minutes and was up against my first challenge in running a household in Africa.

In plenty of time for supper, an American couple came by to welcome us and bring a hot meal and a jug of water, boiled and filtered. Before they departed, they said that if we heard soft rustling sounds in the night, a cobra or some other snake might have made its way inside. Then they offered the helpful information that they kept a pet mongoose to handle any such intruders.

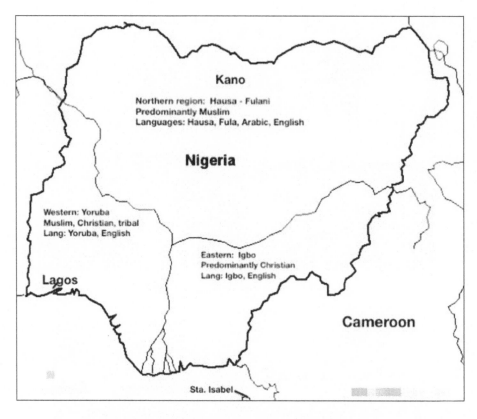

Nigeria's land area: twice the size of California. 1969 Population: 56 million. Tribes: more than 250. Four major tribes constitute 70% of the population. The Hausa and Fulani are often linked together because they are similar and welded together by Islam. Languages/dialects: more than 500, including Nigerian Pidgin. Official language: English

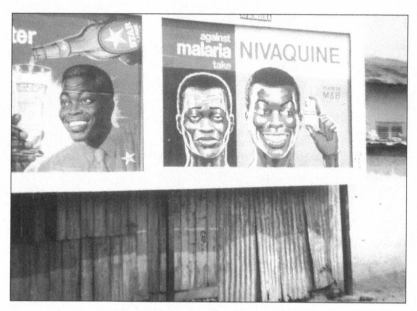

Billboard in Kano, Nigeria, 1969

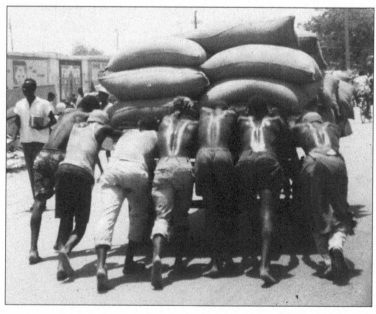

Transporting groundnuts to market, Kano, Nigeria, 1969

# 4

# ADAMU

*During spouses' training* in Atlanta, I'd paid little attention to the session on hiring and managing household help since that wouldn't apply to me. Having servants was so pretentious. Besides, I disliked having to be "on" and interacting with other people all day. I could handle everything myself. So no servants for me, thank you.

I should have paid attention to the training. Africans resented Europeans—they referred to all white people as Europeans—who refused to provide jobs. They viewed us all as rich. If we lived in their country we were obligated to hire their people.

So what to do about Adamu? Carl and I sat on the handmade "Danish" couch to discuss it, and I found myself vigorously swinging one leg, my little nervous habit. I said that with Adamu's winning smile and personality he would have no difficulty finding some other employer. Carl said he'd leave the decision with me, but thought that given the local feelings on the matter, we should probably hire one person.

Ah. There was the rub. You couldn't hire just one. Elaborate etiquette governs the hierarchical structure of Hausa society, and this extends to servants. Each man—all servants were male—did one kind of work. Most refused to do work beneath their level, and they expected an employer to hire others to assist them.

Gardeners were below the in-house hierarchy, but among house servants the ladder's bottom rung belonged to the *small boy*, said with the emphasis on the word small. He scrubbed floors, took out the garbage, did the most unpleasant clean-ups, and served as errand boy for the servants above him in the pecking order. On the next rung up was the laundry man, and above him, the steward. The steward kept the house functional, clean, and in order, with help from the small boy. A cook, who sometimes was a trained chef, sat proud, and often self-important, on the top rung. The caution to hire only men of the same tribe was, of course, not important since I wouldn't be hiring in-house staff.

A guard was a different matter. USAID provided a night watchman, and given the stories we'd heard in Lagos, we did not hesitate to pay for a daytime guard. We hired Musa. He was a Bouzou, the Hausa word for slave. The Bouzou historically, and sometimes today, served as slaves to the elite in the Tuareg bonded servants system. These fierce Berber peoples, both Tuareg and Bouzou, were often dubbed "the blue men," because indigo robes and veils stained their skin. Documentaries and desert movies tell their stories, factual and fanciful.

At five-foot-three, I was almost eye to eye with Musa, but his piercing steel gaze, ramrod-straight bearing and hair-trigger spring in his sandal-clad step dominated his surroundings. A dagger sometimes flashed on his left upper arm. A scimitar hung below his waist on the right. We heard other weaponry was hidden in the folds of his robes. Seasoned Kano residents assured us that while a Bouzou was on duty we would have no thievery, and they warned us that not telling Musa in advance when guests were expected, could lead to tragedy.

I'm glad Musa is here to guard the place, but no other employees please.

*What? What do you mean I'll have to buy chickens live and clucking? And do our laundry on a washboard?* When reality hit, I realized I'd be working as hard as grandmother did on the farm."

Our steward, Adamu—yes, we hired him—could do basic cooking. A former employer of his had taught him to prepare several American dishes, so we paid Adamu more than the standard wage and did not hire a cook. Besides, Adamu ironed clothes. A cook would never stoop so low.

I tried to tell myself I relented on the issue of hiring for altruistic reasons. But I eventually, well, rather quickly, actually, hired Adamu for unvarnished self-preservation.

# 5

# THE LEPERS

*Another American wife* offered to introduce me to the British grocery store, Kingsway. Our primary mission was to buy Dettol dis-
infectant, and my new friend said to buy several liters because
we'd use a lot of it. When we arrived, we found the store's food
inventory was depleted, and the next shipment wasn't due for
another day or two. But besides the Dettol, I did pick up a couple
of other things new to me—Nido powdered milk and Horlicks
Drinking Powder. My English neighbor claimed that Horlicks
mixed with warm milk at bedtime was an excellent sleep aid.

But what I will always remember about the day was the scene
outside the store.

At the entrance were ten or twelve lepers. As soon as we
pulled in, they seemed to call up some hidden strength to move
their bodies to our car. They crowded against the door so that it
was hard to get out. I kept reminding myself of what CDC told
us—unless you're in repeated close personal contact with a person with leprosy, you don't need to be afraid of touching or being
touched. Still, it seemed a little freaky.

Some of the lepers were blind. All had lesions on their ears,
noses and mouths, and some features were misshapen or eat-
en away. Their bodies had large powdery white areas, lesions

everywhere and missing limbs. A leper can lose feeling in the extremities, so without knowing it they get scrapes, cuts and burns. These get infected and tissue dies. Then cartilage gets reabsorbed so the limbs shorten. When a limb becomes infected, gangrene can set in. Next comes amputation. Some men were missing a few fingers or toes, or a hand or foot—others an entire arm or leg. But the most gut-wrenching sight that day at a Western supermarket in Africa were the men who had one or two limbs left, or maybe even just a couple of stumps. They had no way to hold coins or begging bowls, so they rocked their torsos back and forth to scoot their bowls along the ground in front of them.

The more fortunate lepers in Kano State were receiving treatment in Sudan Interior Mission's leprosarium many miles outside the city.

Never much of a jewelry person, I was especially thankful I had none on this day. I could not have felt more inadequate, more helpless, as I gave out my handful of shillings to the men in front of Kingsway. It wasn't enough. It could never be enough.

## Reflection

man with begging bowl—scooting—
scraping on sand
dermis sloughing—adding to sand

how long isolated from others human
how long since he knew he too is human

where shelter these men
where shelter the women
oh, the double misfortune to be leper and woman

# 6

## ‚KANO CITY

*Tom Antorietto, a* short wiry guy with curly black hair and thick,
black-rimmed glasses, checked in with us each day to see how
we were settling in. He'd have clipboard and forms in hand: the
inventory of all the US government furniture in the house, the
list of on-loan linens we could use until our air shipment arrived,
and the list of staple food items placed in the house to welcome
us. I don't remember whether we were to pay for those or replace
them. Did we need additional transformers for our 110-volt appli-
ances? Was there any small appliance we needed to borrow? Tom
was with an Ohio University group and was the USAID business
manager here in Kano. He would make sure all was functional in
our new home.

Today he was at our screen door earlier than usual. With the
meager rainy season at an end, he wanted to get started ahead of
the heat. And before human activity kicked up more dust. The
four of us piled into Tom's car and headed out on a get-acquaint-
ed tour of the city.

My initial impression was once again confirmed—a water-
colorist had come through here with a broad brush and painted
Kano and the countryside with a wash of dusty beige, a wash that
lightened as it climbed into the almost-white sky. Mud houses

and once-white buildings wore the same wash, while burnished black skin and smiles splashing ivory on ebony punctuated the beige. Most of the men—there were few women on the streets—wore robes of white or pale blue and a white kufi, a short fez-style cap, plain or covered with intricate embroidery. Mysterious men robed and veiled in solid indigo, like Musa, were exclamation marks against the bleached backdrop. Just like scenes in desert movies.

Tom broke into my reverie to tell us that Africans were the ultimate recyclers. When those flowing robes wore out, the intact parts of them could be made into smaller items of clothing. When those wore out, smaller pieces or strips of the cloth could serve a variety of other purposes. There seemed to be nothing that could not be recycled. You could even say that these mud houses were recycled. What to do when weather wears away your house? Use remaining mud to start a new house. If not enough mud for that, make earthen ovens. When walls and ovens disintegrate, take the mud and make earthen pots.

Tom showed us the way to the central market. He introduced us to the bookstore, the stationery store, and the Bata store with its Spanish-made shoes.

Inside the dusty post office, we bought postage stamps from a man losing his battle with a particularly zealous fly. The sticky yellow flypaper hanging from the ceiling already hosted a capacity crowd. We checked out the telecommunications area. Tom indicated a wooden desk and the uniformed man we would work with to place a telephone call. International calls required advance scheduling, and the phone booths and a row of wooden chairs were filling with customers who had scheduled calls the day before. Callers shouted into the big heavy-looking phones.

At Barclays Bank we exchanged dollars for Nigerian pounds

and shillings and got our first taste of stiff bureaucratic English and the webs of red tape the Nigerians had learned so thoroughly from their colonial "masters." The syncopated clunk-swish-clunk of rubber stamp after rubber stamp made American bureaucracy look spare.

Tom advised us on how to take care of business in Kano. He said a lot of palaver—lengthy discussion—was required to accomplish anything. He explained the *dash*, both the noun and the verb. "To get things done you have to expect to *dash* an official by slipping him a *dash*. Da-shee, da-shee." Apparently, nothing could untangle a snarl of red tape like the dash.

Adding his own horn to the din of bicycle bells and truck horns, Tom maneuvered his big American car—Chevrolet, I think—through the now-packed streets. I called Charles's attention to a man carrying a tall glass bottle on his head. "Kerosene," Tom said. Kerosene? In that tall, skinny bottle? On his head?

Colorful enameled pans full of spices and foods for sale, and every household item imaginable, appeared everywhere, balanced on heads of pedestrians and even bicyclists. Head-bearing was obviously the preferred means of carrying any item, no matter the size. A tightly wrapped fabric donut placed on the head created a level base and steadied the item. But I could hardly believe it when I saw a man, his gait and posture smooth and aristocratic, bearing on his head a full-sized, cabinet-style treadle sewing machine.

The encyclopedia had said that historically Africans liked to keep their hands free in case of an emergency, such as the need to fend off an enemy or a wild animal attack. That must explain such perfect posture.

We made a brief stop in the hospital's crowded parking lot, and Tom pointed out the main and emergency entrances. He described the check-in procedure and reminded us to always bring our own disposable syringes and needles. On advice from CDC we had brought a good supply of those in our air shipment.

Tom made a quick stop at a store to buy a case of the sugary, syrupy *Squash* that's a staple beverage in a lot of expat kitchens. His boys loved it, and some English children refused to drink anything else. It was rumored to have a little fruit juice, but I personally don't think fruit had come within a mile of it. I spotted the colorful jars of Marmite the English are so crazy about. It's a sticky brown spread, very salty, a byproduct of beer brewing. My neighbor from Britain said you either hate it or you love it. I read the label. Pretty sure I'd be in the "hate it" camp.

Away from the central area and its shops, we drove along the railroad tracks to view rows and rows of Kano pyramids, a major tourist attraction in West Africa. They were the wealth of the area—groundnuts (peanuts).

During the harvest, heavy bags of groundnuts were brought into Kano by donkey, camel, truck or flat-bed cart pushed by five or six men. Deposited on a field along the railroad tracks, about 15,000 bags went into a single pyramid. Placement of the final and topmost bag of a pyramid called for celebration. Everyone left work and turned out to watch. These magnificent structures began to appear each fall and grew until they dwarfed the buildings in Kano. They grew smaller and eventually disappeared as the bags were shipped to Lagos by rail.

We passed the central mosque and the high mud walls of the palace of Emir Ado Bayero, the Islamic spiritual leader for Kano and surrounding villages. Just as we drove past, the emir, or at least his car, was driving away from the palace. I got a blurry photo of the pale aqua-blue Rolls Royce Queen Elizabeth had ridden in when she visited Nigeria.

It was hot by the time we arrived at the indigo dye pits, but for at least ten minutes we stood in the sun, feet escaping through strappy sandals into burning sand, and watched men repeatedly plunge fabric into the dye made from indigo plants grown just outside the city. Tom told us the men sometimes continued for hours plunging and wringing and plunging again. Between wiping dust from the corners of my eyes, I kept winding my 8mm camera to record this ancient art of tie-dye. Each one of dozens of circular pits in the ground had been passed from father to son since 1498.

I drank up all these new sights and sounds. Oh, the thrill of experiencing a new culture! My romanticized idea of Africa was confirmed and enhanced with each new adventure, but I discovered that half a day was enough to be out and about here at the edge of the Sahel. As I cooled down with a tall glass of iced tea, I realized I hadn't asked Tom anything about the war. Didn't Dr. Arnold say that Kano had been a flash point for the Nigerian Civil War? I needed to ask Tom about that.

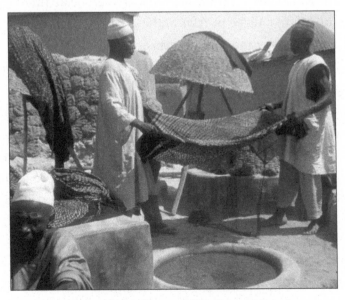

Dye pits dating from 1498, Kano, Nigeria

# 7

# SMALLPOX TARGET ZERO

*If I had* been caught off guard to find a servant already installed at our house, Carl had been even more caught off guard. He arrived at his post in Kano to find his counterpart missing.

At training in Atlanta, each operations officer was partnered with the person who would serve as their native counterpart once they arrived in Africa. It was a brilliant plan. The two would go through the same training and also have social time together while in Atlanta. Once in Africa, the getting-to-know-you period wouldn't have so many false starts and detours.

Carl's assigned counterpart was Malam Kazari, *Malam* being a respectful form of address like Mr., for an educated man or an Islamic teacher. We had enjoyed lots of evenings with him at our apartment. We shared meals, and he shared stories and photographs of Kano. He often showed up an hour late for dinner and sometimes brought along uninvited guests. We were told to expect that in Africa, so we learned to prepare extra food just in case. Once, I even tried to prepare an African dinner for him. I don't know what I was thinking.

One weekend, I went with M. Kazari to downtown Atlanta to help him shop for things to take home to Nigeria. I was embarrassed at the horrified glares from other shoppers. A white woman together with a black man—choosing bedding and bath linens no less! It reminded me of the times Carl and I had gone on outings with his African fellow students in Houston. Seven years later, in Atlanta, not much had changed.

But back to the missing Malam. He had arrived in Kano three weeks ahead of us and used his CDC training certificate to move on to a more prestigious job. We had to be happy for him, but what a setback for Carl—to start with an unknown counterpart and one who hadn't been through the same training. Typical for Carl though, he didn't let this delay his start by much.

At least the vaccinators on his team, about twelve Nigerians, had worked with his predecessor for a year or more. Carl was impressed with their work, even from those who'd had no opportunity to go beyond a primary education.

I wrote our family a long letter:

> Hello, dear ones!
>
> I can't believe we'll have to content ourselves with letters and may not hear your voices for two whole years! Letters may take up to four weeks to reach you.
>
> We're sort of settled into our house. Didn't take long because all we have is the air shipment. There's no telling how many ports of call our sea shipment will visit before it reaches Lagos. It'll take weeks to clear customs and then be trucked to Kano. We won't see it for a few months yet I'm sure. AID people here outfitted the house with loaner dishes, pots and pans, bedding and a few basic food items to help us get through the first few days.
>
> Since eradicating smallpox, and controlling measles too, is the reason we're here, and since you always want to know how Carl spends his day, I'll try to give you a crash course—on smallpox. Well, okay, a few basics. WHO's

end goal is zero pox, as in zero pox in the entire world! Can you imagine? That means not only *variola major* (kills about thirty percent of victims) but also *variola minor* (kills about three percent) because of the fear that *variola minor* may mutate into more of a killer.

The global campaign starts with these nineteen countries in the West and Central Africa program. And— because measles is such a child-killer in West Africa (anywhere from a twenty percent to a fifty percent death rate), these countries pushed to have measles control included in the program.

I knew that some family members would want a lot more detail than others, but it was too time consuming to write separate accounts. I put all the information I could and left it to each person to read or skim as they desired.

The old feudal system is still in place up here in Muslim northern Nigeria, so much so that it feels in some ways like traveling back to the Middle Ages. But that has great advantages for the smallpox program because the emirs direct people to get vaccinated. Since people seldom disobey the emir, Carl doesn't face the resistance to vaccination that faces some of his colleagues.

People who practice some of the tribal religions believe the Yoruba god Shapona causes, and cures, smallpox, and that humans must not interfere. They hide an infected person. And because witchdoctors' and fetishers' influence and income are threatened by getting rid of the disease, they warn people against vaccination, and sometimes even threaten to spread smallpox.

But on to what the work is like for Carl. I hope you can picture him out there—in the bush or in the city.

For the mass vaccination campaigns, assembly points are set up (selected so people don't have to walk farther than 8 km to reach the site), and the vaccinators and their jet injectors go to work. Smallpox vaccination is given to everyone, and measles vaccination to young children.

In these Muslim areas, they vaccinate men and women separately. The men go through the line first and then go home and bring the women and children. I'm trying to picture families who live several kilometers away. Do the men bring the women and stash them out of sight somewhere, get themselves vaccinated and then go retrieve the women from hiding?

The Ped-O-Jet (jet injector) looks like a gun with two tubes hanging from it and a bottle of vaccine sitting on top. The air hose connects it to a foot pedal. When the vaccinator pumps the pedal, a regulated dose of vaccine penetrates the skin by speed and force. No needle! That's for me! They can vaccinate a thousand people an hour. In one campaign here in Nigeria, in only ten days twelve teams and an army of volunteers vaccinated more than 750,000 people.

The first teams came out here two years ago (1967) and have completed most of the mass smallpox vaccination campaign. Carl and the others still use that strategy for measles, but for most of the smallpox vaccinations, CDC has switched to a newer approach, developed by Dr. Foege. It's called surveillance and containment or the ring method. They go everywhere, show the smallpox identification photo and ask, "Have you seen anyone who looks like this?" They hold publicity campaigns, and in areas where it's hard to convince people to get vaccinated, they host festive events—anything to make it attractive and keep the smallpox fight front and center in people's minds. They offer rewards for identifying a case of smallpox.

When one case is found, everything happens fast. First, immediate quarantine. Then the teams descend on the area to vaccinate or revaccinate all the patient's contacts. And—the contacts of *those* contacts. Just like in fighting a forest fire they build a firewall around the virus to contain the outbreak. It's a real race against the clock. Carl's record-setting contact tracing skill is definitely needed out here in Africa. (Are you bragging on your son yet, Mom?)

Because of the speed of moving from one place to another, even one house to another, they use the bifurcated (two-pronged) needle rather than the Ped-O-Jet. Besides the obvious advantages, it uses less vaccine, and in fifteen minutes they can teach volunteers how to use it.

Carl says some of his CDC colleagues think it's risky to switch from mass vaccination to surveillance and containment, and a few grumble about the change. But the approach seems to have proven itself. He's sold on it, especially when his teams have to vaccinate in widely scattered villages or need to intercept nomads on the move. Contact tracing and all aspects of battling a virus are especially daunting tasks among any mobile population.

CDC listens to anyone with a new idea of how to improve the campaign and then tests those ideas. They told us they recruited men and women who are flexible and adaptable. People who will quickly change course as methods, migrations, weather or local rulers change. Carl fits that description in spades.

Congratulations! You've finished Smallpox Lesson 1.

Now for Lesson 2.

If you'd like to know how people inoculated against smallpox before discovery of the vaccine, what do you think of this method? Way back in history, the Chinese took dried smallpox scabs, ground them to powder, and blew the powder up a person's nose to inoculate him.

Then, in the early 1700s, people here in West Africa, and also in Turkey, took infected material from a smallpox sore and inserted it just into the skin of a well person for the same purpose—to cause a, hopefully, very light case of smallpox and consequently, life-long immunity. Since this and the powder-up-the-nose method were with the actual smallpox virus (variolation), about one person out of a hundred came down with a full-blown case, some fatal. So you can imagine that the resistance to its use included death threats, even though those odds were far better than the one in three from naturally acquired smallpox.

How this method made it to the English court and across the pond to Boston is a fascinating story but too long for my letter. You might want to check your Britannica. Look up these four names and you'll find the whole story: Lady Mary Wortley Montagu, Cotton Mather, Doctor Zabdiel Boylston, and Onesimus, an African slave.

Then the life-saving breakthrough!! Vaccine!! Developed half a century later by Dr. Edward Jenner. (Another great story to look up in your encyclopedia.) Vaccine is infinitely safer as it doesn't put smallpox into the body. Obviously, our teams try to educate any fetishers who practice variolation. It does put smallpox into the body.

Just one more bit of history. Abraham Lincoln was not

at all well when he delivered the Gettysburg Address, and a couple of days later, he developed the rash. Smallpox. He was kept secluded in the White House for the next ten days. (His personal valet later came down with smallpox and died.) If his incubation period had been two days shorter, we might not have had those famous words.

This concludes your smallpox lesson. Be ready for a pop quiz. Ha.

I miss all of you, but I am so excited to be here. I know Carl is going to help make history. The Hausa people have been warm and welcoming, and the handful of American families here with USAID are glad to see some new faces. Every single day I have a new experience. Some are grim and tough to take. I wasn't prepared for the sight of small-pox survivors who have deep disfiguring scars covering every inch, or lepers' unimaginable deformities. I hope I don't get so used to the sight of suffering I become jaded.

I have to close for now. My English neighbor across the road is "calling on me" in a few minutes. I'll not embarrass myself by trying to serve an English tea. We hope you're all well, and please, please write soon.

Big hugs to everyone,

Bee

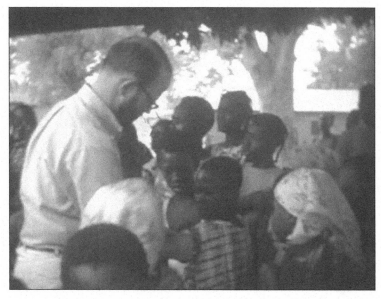

Carl checking for smallpox scars in a Nigerian village, 1969

# 8

## MANGOES AND MAMBAS

*Morning in Nigeria* began with the jingle of bicycle bells as the smell of charcoal cooking fires and a succession of traders arrived at our door. Each vendor offered a different specialty—bread, green vegetables and potatoes, mangoes, groundnuts, eggs and chickens. We tested the eggs for freshness with a pan of water. The fresher the egg, the more horizontal it lies on the bottom. I refused any egg that assumed a vertical posture, especially if it bobbed up and peeked at me over the surface of the water.

Except for the egg inspection, which I had fun doing, Adamu handled most food purchases. He was expert at getting the best prices. Those live chickens weren't clucking as they hung by their ankles from bicycle handlebars. An occasional squawk maybe. Adamu knew how to choose a young, tender one. He checked for bright feathers, and bright, not faded, colors of beak, comb and earlobes.

Earlobes! A chicken has earlobes?

It turns out they do. And who knew white-earlobed hens lay white eggs, and red ear-lobed hens lay brown or speckled eggs?

Adamu could expertly select the best local mangoes, avoiding the ones that smelled of kerosene. All mangoes naturally contain some kerosene, and one of Kano's local varieties was even named *kerosene mango*. Still, best to follow the rule: if you can smell it, discard it.

While dealing with the vendors, Adamu also bought food for his own family, often including chili peppers. Having lived in New Mexico, I considered myself a fire eater. So much so that I had packed a large container of the addictive chilies in our air shipment. I was thrilled to discover a producing chili plant outside our back door. As I plucked one, Adamu tried to stop me.

"Oh, madame! This for African. European cannot eat."

I thanked Adamu but told him not to worry about me. "I love chilies and eat them all the time." *This* European could handle chilies just fine.

He tried one more time, insisting this chili was not like in America.

Poor Adamu. He just didn't get it, but it was sweet of him to try to protect me.

I took one bite. After the intense heat came a strong and pungent taste. Too late. Borderline nausea followed the pain. European, indeed, cannot eat. I catch on fast.

Despite our dry air here near the Sahara, the kitchen was humidified by the nonstop boiling of water. We had to stave off the threat of amoebic dysentery with its violent diarrhea, cramps, chills and fever. The amoeba parasite hid behind the next sip of water or bite of food. (It can travel to the liver and can even be life threatening.)

The amenities paragraph in the booklet *Kano State* touts electricity and "pipe-borne water." This more-precious-than-gold liquid was delivered to a three-foot-diameter tank on the roof. Gravity delivered it to the taps, which is where our work began—Adamu's work to be precise. After a twenty-minute rolling boil, the water made a slow trip through the "candle filter," a ceramic pillar the shape of a two-inch-diameter candle inside the tall Royal Doulton crock on our kitchen counter. We could now draw safe water from the crock's spigot and put the next pot on to boil. We needed enough safe water to drink, make ice for iced tea, cook, wash hands and faces and brush teeth.

(Despite the inconvenience of fending off waterborne diseases, it was nothing compared to a daily one- or two-hour walk just to get water, often at a contaminated source, experienced by many in sub-Saharan Africa. Then add hauling the water home and storing it. The hauling and storing made it vulnerable to contamination even if it had been safe at the source. And how many children had no opportunity for schooling because of the hours spent hauling water! So our boiling and filtering was more of a First-World problem than you might at first think.)

Our fruits and vegetables were rendered safe to eat by a twenty-minute soak in a mixture of one part bleach to ten parts of the processed water. I never learned to like the limp lettuce, post bleach-water soak.

But that wasn't the end of the food-and-drink safety measures. We washed down the kitchen counter with Clorox or Dettol before all food preparation tasks. The area behind the counters, the wall behind the counters, the sink, cutting boards, knives, kitchen gloves and table got their bleach bath as well. With bravado, some Americans ridiculed the more vigilant of us. Given Carl's work with disease and disease prevention, and his watchfulness when it came to his family, we were in the vigilant camp. I could say we had the last laugh, but no one laughed when someone came down with "the amoeba."

We always had a supply of frozen food because we were assigned a freezer for the measles vaccine. In earlier days, keeping measles vaccine viable in the bush had been a challenge. Now

Carl took out the amount of vaccine needed each day. The teams then placed it into kerosene-powered refrigerators mounted on the trucks, thus maintaining "the cold chain."

One day I heard excited sounds coming from the kitchen. Adamu had asked the kids if they liked peanut butter. He shelled and roasted fresh groundnuts, and then rolled them with a glass jar to crush and grind them to a smooth and crunchy golden perfection. A bit of salt finished the irresistible treat.

Adamu did all this and more, smile still intact, and somewhere along the way found time to wring the neck of that chicken and get it plucked, cleaned and cooked.

For safety at night, Adamu lined our drive with lanterns—empty food cans punched with holes in attractive patterns, tallow and a wick in the bottom. When a lantern or some other empty-can repurposed item got too old or damaged, Nigerians cut them into triangles or other shapes to use as decoration or reflectors hung in the sun to repel flies.

Audu, our small boy, was hire number three—don't laugh—after Musa and Adamu. Audu was short and slender, and at about twenty years of age, he was glad to learn a new skill to increase his income and future work prospects. We taught him to wash clothes. At best, he had a half-hearted relationship with the washboard and didn't hide his delight when USAID bought us a wringer washing machine.

Identical to the one Grandmother used on the farm in the '40s, the round-bottomed tub perched high on its wheeled legs in a corner of the kitchen. It could be rolled to the sink where one hose connected to the faucet and the other, for draining, hooked over the edge of the sink. Audu learned the hard way to keep fingers at a safe distance while feeding clothes in between the two rollers. Out on the clothesline, washed clothes dried to brittle sheets within minutes. Adamu sprayed these dry wafers with water or starch and ironed them.

And then there was the water-related issue of bath time. Lathering and then rinsing one body quadrant at a time was a strategic adaptation to avoid having a completely lathered body when there was suddenly no water.

Most days began with water in the roof tank, but laundry day stressed the supply. On the no-water mornings, laundry and baths had to get in line behind the water headed to the huge pot on the stove. Days with no water at all gave Audu a break from washing and Adamu a break from mopping. (Because of all the dust, Adamu chose to clean the floors two to three times a day.) Other breaks for the men came during power outages or when someone neglected to use the transformers that prevented the 220-volt wiring from burning up our vacuum or some other 110-volt appliance.

When it came to water, electricity, plumbing or anything else about daily life, we followed advice from British and American old-timers around here. "Don't expect things to work and you won't be frustrated. People get exhausted from the hassle, and it's the small frustrations that are the final straw. Relax."

From the beginning, Carl and I had expected things would often not work. In fact, we rather enjoyed the evenings without electricity. With family privacy after Adamu's postdinner departure, we could just break out the candles, sit with Charles and Ginger, and draw, tell stories or play a simple game.

Why we hired a gardener I can't remember, and cannot fathom, because our "yard" was a natural part of the transition from Sahel to savanna, a handful of trees planted years earlier by the British, a half acre of dry dust and scrub and one lone flowering frangipani tree. Perhaps the lack of bushes and irrigation trenches accounted for our having had no nighttime cobra visitations. We had arrived at the end of the June-to-September rainy season, too late to even enjoy the twenty-seven inches of annual rainfall. Shetima, while he was watering, could stand in one spot for more than ten minutes on end, looking off into space. He reminded me of a yard-art fountain sculpture, sending an anemic arc of water from the nozzle onto the same square foot of sponge-thirsty dirt. He appeared not to notice the futility, or care. Still, he validated our decision to hire him. In his pointy knit cap, he came to the door one day with a long dark brown snake, hanging lifeless from the tip of his arrow. With his usual flat expression he explained, "Snake for yard, madame. Black mamba. I shoot."

I didn't have the presence of mind to save the body to show Carl when he came in from the bush. Confirming the kind of snake slithering through one's yard or deciding to start a family in the shade of one's house would be important information. The black mamba moves faster than most humans can run, and its bite is a quick death sentence without antivenom intervention. Whether black mamba or no, Shetima had earned his spot on our payroll. He could water the dry dust all he wanted to.

So, despite my past protests, there we were with the obligatory hierarchy of staff. A retinue of five, if you count the night watchman USAID hired for us. I'd recharge and enjoy my solitude when all the staff left after lunch. On the edge of the Sahel, nothing and nobody moved in the afternoon, so it would be quiet. And only Adamu came back for the dinner hour.

We had followed the dictum to be sure all the servants were of the same tribe, and certainly of the same religion, in the interest of peace. In our house all the men were Muslim, and all except Musa were Hausa. Their temperaments were compatible too. Adamu and Audu were both easygoing, and Audu was the quiet type. Shetima was pleasant enough and seemed happy to be left to daydream and to wander around the property, placid unless venomous visitors came to call. Musa didn't interact with the others. There'd be no palaver with this fierce warrior of the Sahara. Man of few words. None needed.

Adamu laughed with a contagious melody that drew you in. He took delight in the smallest things it seemed. At least he was always smiling. If Carl or I argued or sounded worried, his brow furrowed, his eyes probed, and his head adopted a perplexed tilt to one side. Just how serious was our problem anyway?

I'd like to be him when I grow up.


The men admired our son's creativity in his drawing and his paper-hat making, and they couldn't believe how much he knew. "Oh, you smart man, Mister Charles."

Adamu wrapped turbans around Ginger's head and secured her baby dolls on her back, Africa-style. Our children's faces brightened when Adamu laughed with them or when the men whittled toys for them from a branch from one of the scrub bushes. Adamu's own little girl played in our yard too. Cute and spunky, she was her daddy's delight.

The men on our staff liked Carl, and he liked them. When he was at the house, his next expression of gratitude for even the most minor bit of work was never far off. One of our family members back home was often annoyed by Carl's repeated thank-yous, but the Africans seemed pleased.

I liked each one of the men and was grateful for the work they did. I had plenty to do. We had no TV and no radio, and news magazines were weeks old. I continued to read my speech pathology journals to keep up to date in the profession I had embarked on before we left the States. I enjoyed having time to do crafts with the children, read, cook unfamiliar foods and experience the market trips and other adventures that presented themselves. And I appreciated having someone else kill our dinner.

Oh, all right. I'll keep the servants if you insist.

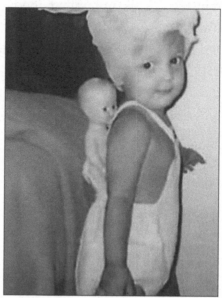

Adamu enjoyed styling Ginger as
an "Africa woman"

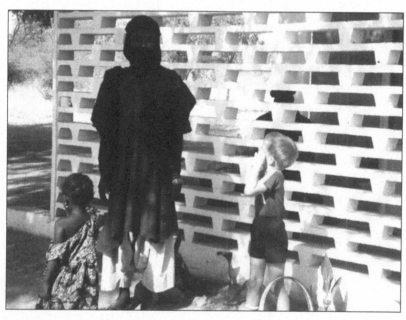

Adamu's daughter, Musa, and Charles at our house in Kano

# 9

# GREEN

*This Saturday morning,* Tom Antorietto was at our screen door again, this time sans clipboard. He said there was something Carl and I should see. If we were available, he would drive us there right then.

On the way, he was unusually quiet. After about ten minutes, he told us to look to our left after the next turn because we were about to pass the saddest site in Kano.

We turned onto a road that hugged the thousand-year-old outer perimeter Old City wall. On our left, at a place where the wall angled away from the road, a flat, bright green patch of land, around ten acres I think, lay in stark relief against the unbroken beige of the African Sahel. The contrast was unexpected, and our questioning looks begged for an explanation.

Tom may not have known what kind of plant formed the verdant carpet, but he knew why it was so green.

As I remember it, Tom's usual slow and soft way of talking unrolled the scene one painful frame at a time. "Mass grave . . . bodies of the Igbo—men, women, children . . . thousands . . . massacred three years ago . . . genocide. Nigerian army started, you know . . . and it wasn't long till angry mobs joined in.

They'll never know how many were killed." In Tom's achingly long pauses, I couldn't speak. Even Carl grew quiet.

We hadn't read TIME magazine's October 1966 report of the event. "When it fought with U.N. forces in the Congo, the Nigerian army's 5th Battalion took special pride in its rigid military discipline," the TIME story said. "That was only three years ago, but as far as Nigeria is concerned, it is the remote past. Last week the 5th's proud tradition collapsed in an orgy of mass savagery that rivaled anything the Congo had ever known . . ."

Tom said the primarily Hausa army started killing Igbos at the Kano airport, continued through the center of town, and then swarmed into the *Sabon Gari* (Strangers' Quarter) with guns and clubs, cutlasses and scimitars, stones and broken glass.

In Kano, and throughout the north, from May through October of '66, many thousands of Igbo were slaughtered, one of the final sparks that detonated the Nigeria-Biafra War. Tom said if we had the stomach for it, we could read the grisly details. Of how the attackers sliced their way through the population. Of what they did to pregnant women, old men, children, everyone. He warned that the mental images would keep us awake at night.

I couldn't begin to process my emotions.

There'd been a series of massacres up here in the north. Almost all the Igbo who could escape left everything. Left their homes. Left their businesses. Tried to get to their homeland in the east. Roads were clogged with bicycles, cars, trucks, people on foot. Many were hacked to pieces on the trains and roads going out of the north.

How could I grapple with what Tom was telling us? I had no framework in which to place it. That exotic National Geographic-like image my mind had created and clutched so tenaciously before our arrival was now nowhere in sight.

———⟩

But the Kano massacre was one in a series of attacks, coups and countercoups since independence from Britain in 1960. As Elaine Neil Orr said in her memoir, *Gods of Noonday: A White Girl's African Life,* "The country was being born and the umbilical cord was wound around its neck like a python."

Sadly, the mass grave outside our car window was not a rarity on a continent where the new countries were fractured from the start. Africa's modern states were forced upon people with nothing in common. At the table and in the back rooms of the Berlin Conference in the late 1800s, the colonial powers had carved up and dished out the African continent to fit their own interests. The unique tribal territories meant nothing to the men at the table. Tribes and clans were ripped apart by lines on a map.

Nearly a century later, as these colonies became independent, rival tribes were thrust under a common government not of their making. Each tribe tried to shore up its power in a "nation" to which it had no allegiance and in which tribal interests were often mutually exclusive. Fierce tribal rivalries that the colonial powers had kept under control, even while exploiting those rivalries, often flared into violent conflict.

One in five sub-Saharan Africans lived in Nigeria. Under colonial rule it had been two countries—Northern Nigeria and Southern Nigeria—until the British stapled the two parts together. Their policies favored the north because the Islamic emirates' feudal system suited England's practice of indirect rule. The emirs collected taxes for England, and England obstructed the entrance of Christian missionaries into the Islamic north.

But despite Britain's favors to the Hausa-Fulani, the Igbo had landed responsible jobs throughout Nigeria. They doggedly pursued education and business, and large numbers had migrated to the north, where they owned businesses or held prominent government positions. With the 1966 massacres, as many as thirty thousand (by some estimates vastly more) of those migrants would not leave the north alive.

And tribal conflicts? They reached into the distant past, long before colonization. I was looking out the window at an artifact of history, something that might be documented in dry summary on a page somewhere.

But looking at this green, it was too immediate. Words deserted me.

→

On May 30, 1967, eight months after the bloody pogrom, Colonel Odumegwu Ojukwu had declared the southeastern corner of Nigeria to be the Republic of Biafra. Fear of genocide, but also the discovery of oil in the southeast, had fueled the secessionist movement. In the war that followed, an estimated 100,000 were killed in combat. Journalists reporting from inside Biafra witnessed an army practicing with wooden "guns." In battle, they witnessed young boys fighting barefoot. And often, with one gun for each two soldiers, as one was killed the other took over the gun. The Nigerian federal government imposed an air, land and sea blockade, and as a result, up to two million Biafrans died of disease and starvation, despite clandestine nighttime relief flights from nearby islands such as Fernando Po.

War or no war, our campaign could not slow its pace if the world was ever to be free of smallpox. Even during the bitter conflict, brief cease-fires were arranged to allow transfer of vaccine into Biafra and specimens from suspected smallpox cases out of

Biafra to a laboratory in Lagos. The full global campaign to eradicate smallpox would encompass a decade. It would push through other wars before the last case was diagnosed.

—➤

Looking back, it all seems surreal. Arriving in August of 1969, we didn't notice the war. During our family's orientation week in bustling Lagos, I heard nobody speak of war. Dinner parties were illuminated by Japanese lanterns and worldly conversation. Out and about, few military uniforms were to be seen. Stores were fully stocked and full of shoppers. University students prepared for exams.

Tom had a shortwave radio in his office at Kano Teachers College, where he and his fellow Ohio University advisors worked. If he listened to war reports on the BBC World Service or the Voice of America, I didn't hear about it. And—we had no television. We saw no images. None of the heart-rending photographs of starving Biafran children the rest of the world saw. Life and commerce went on. It was indeed the "staggering normalcy" that Harry Reasoner talked about.

The only trace of war here in Kano was this expanse of green.

—➤

We couldn't know then that five decades later, after more cycles of hate and war, many new mass graves would interrupt the beige landscape of this same African savanna and Sahel. That a group called Boko Haram would be born and, in atrocities not reserved for Christians or for Igbo, would massacre fellow Muslims, "infidels" not adhering to their exclusive beliefs. Hausa or Fulani friends we made in Kano, their children or grandchildren—would they themselves be among the victims? And, terrible as it is to ask, would some join the hordes who continue the cycles of violence?

Looking at this mass grave, we couldn't know that in 2015 a girl would appear in school uniform at Kano Teachers College and detonate the bombs hidden under her uniform, taking dozens of lives along with her own.

With the patch of green in our rearview mirror, Tom turned at the next corner. As we headed in the direction of our oleander-hedged neighborhood, I somehow felt older than I'd felt mere minutes before.

# 10

# TECHNOLOGY 1969

*I wouldn't be* able to call my sister and tell her about the horrors of the mass grave.

If I wanted to make a phone call, I would have to go to the phone center at the post office and book the call a day ahead. The cost would be prohibitive.

All our communications were limited.

Carl could go to Tom's office at Kano Teachers College when he needed to communicate, securely or not, with the CDC in Atlanta or with his program's regional office in Lagos. If I remember correctly, these communications did not include telephone.

News from home, or from anywhere outside Kano, was slow in coming. We had no radio. Letters either to or from the States could be a month or more in transit. We discontinued newspaper and magazine subscriptions when we moved to Africa. Our friends who didn't received news that was weeks or months old.

Cell phones and the internet were years in the future.

# 11

# SMALLPOX/MEASLES LOGISTICS

*I had never* been good about keeping in touch by mail, but here in Africa I made the effort. Especially when it came to reassuring Carl's parents—"Please don't worry about us, we're fine, really, we're fine, well and happy, fine. We're fine."

I'd think of local color things that might take their minds off worrying about us. Things like the termite hills, those rusty spires that are such a prominent feature of the bush landscape, their height reflecting the depth of the colony's chambers since they're formed by the excavated earth. Some hills are more than twenty feet high—the New York Cities of the termite world. The spires become hard clay, great scratching posts for cattle and camels. Or I'd offer minutiae like the fact that in this climate and this kind of fieldwork, Carl had long since given up wearing his turquoise bolo tie.

The more I could tell the family about day-to-day life in Africa and about Carl's work, the better. Like how he had to plan when and where to vaccinate based on Muslim prayer time and mosque days, severe dust storms blowing off the Sahara, and seasonal migration of nomads and their flocks. Those migrations were a critical factor because they could reintroduce the virus in an area that had been freed of smallpox.

Or I could tell them about Carl's driver, Meninge, who was also his interpreter. Although English is the official language in Nigeria and used by people who've had easy access to education, others communicate in native languages and dialects, or in pidgin English, a language created from elements of their dialect and elements of English. (There are variations of pidgin all over the world.) Northern Nigeria alone has dozens of native dialects. And because the Hausa and the Fulani are Muslim, many also speak Arabic. Meninge could handle most language challenges as well as those of road and truck.

In letters to my own parents or my sister, I could "fess up" about more of the challenges:

> I have to tell you about our trucks. Oh my goodness. Parts and maintenance. What a problem! You see, USAID requires us to use American-made vehicles. CDC tried to get an exemption for working in this environment but no such luck. The huge Dodge Power Wagon is too wide for a lot of the roads and is too heavy for the bridges. In other parts of West Africa, many bridges are made of bamboo and our trucks often break through!
>
> Breakdowns happen out in the bush all the time. You should see the line of seven or eight trucks broken down awaiting repair. It's a smallpox program salvage yard. When an axle snaps, they might have to wait at least two months for one to be shipped from the States. Or it could be longer. The Vietnam War has priority. Some trucks are cannibalized to provide parts for others. In areas where there are rubber trees, repairs might be rigged with tree sap and cotton balls!
>
> We need vehicles suited to Africa—with fuel filters

that tolerate the local gasoline, with availability of local parts and service. Not a truck too wide, too heavy, too everything for the environment. In other words, we need Land Rovers. Next month Carl and all the other operations officers go to Ghana, for two weeks I think he said, to learn basic truck maintenance. You know what a stretch that'll be for Carl. Can you just picture it?

And speaking of repairs, those Ped-O-Jets that are so critical to mass vaccination are often out of commission— dust clogging the nozzles and precision workings. CDC taught repair of those while we were in Atlanta.

For letters to Mom and Pop (Carl's parents), bragging on him and his work was always an acceptable topic:

Carl loves what he's doing! The army of people, up and down the chain, are great to work with. The Atlanta program managers hired people they believed to be creative and independent—so they leave them alone to do the job. Out here, the guys can't just pick up a phone and call Lagos or Atlanta if there's a problem. Carl is thriving with the freedom to resolve issues in the field, on the spot.

He does get on a soapbox (you know how he can do that) about the need for an integrated approach to development, with education, agriculture and transportation concurrent with health initiatives, including clean water.

He says I can go to the field with him sometime when a whole team of Muslim men is not going. It's nice he sometimes takes Charles to the field with him.

Each day is an adventure here, even if it's only in the kitchen or going to eat at the Kano Club. That's an interesting outing, especially when we see any of the British "old Africa hands." I'll write about the club another time.

Oh, yes. I want to close with one final word about smallpox. The operations manual emphasizes to always defer to the local ministries of health, to be sure any publicity campaign puts the spotlight on them, and to give them the credit for everything that's accomplished, but just between us, you'd be so proud of Carl.

Then I'd sign off the letter with more assurances that we were fine.

The family didn't know how skilled Carl was. Or how tough. As a venereal disease (VD) investigator, he'd worked the streets armed with interview and investigation techniques designed by the FBI. He was the best around at contact tracing—finding who had given the disease to his subject case and who his subject may have passed it on to. "Source and Spread" they called it.

Whether he was hunting down contacts in rural Arkansas, the streets of New York City or Albuquerque or across the Navajo, Hopi and Zuni reservations, it was critical to find every possible case or at-risk person and get them treated with penicillin.

Carl wasn't typically greeted with, "Oh, you're from the health department here to ask about my sex life? Come on in. Can I get you a cup of coffee?" Even to get a person to come to the door, he sometimes had to be as wily as a process server.

Once he did get a conversation going, not everyone was eager to share the names of all the people they'd had sex with—sometimes hundreds. When they didn't know last names, or even first names, such contacts would be *unk-unk* (unknown-unknown). Then Carl had to dig for bits and pieces—physical description, where a person hung out, where they worked, hobbies, habits. Anything at all.

The VD "case" Carl was interviewing might only know the contact was a stranger met in a bar. Sometimes a caller rang our phone in the middle of the night saying, "You know that person you needed to find? Well he's (or she's) here right now at the such-and-such bar." Then Carl got out of bed, took his dark-field microscope and his wits and went to the such-and-such bar.

Now Carl and a number of his fellow VD investigators applied their contact-tracing skills to the contagion of smallpox. With a passion.

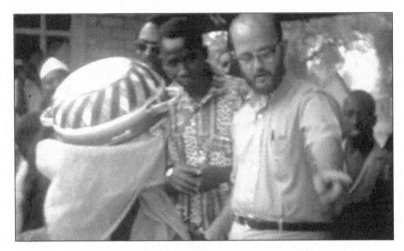

Carl on the job

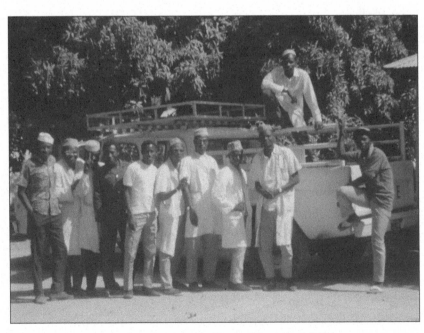

Vaccination team, Kano, Nigeria, 1970

# 12

# THE MOON AND MAN

*Our screen door* banged shut as Carl hurried in, out of breath, lugging a Bell & Howell projector and a 16mm film canister. "Bee, hurry and set up the movie screen. My team members are on their way here."

I knew Carl was working in the city today, not out in the bush, but he never came home midmorning except to get more vaccine from the freezer. What was this about? Another training?

No, not a training. He said most of the guys on his teams didn't believe we landed on the moon. "I went to the USIS library for a film on the space program. Might make it seem more real."

We had arrived in Nigeria six weeks after the first moon landing. The "alleged" event had been widely talked about in town, and for good reason. At the beginning of space travel, NASA installed orbital tracking stations around the globe. The last one was completed in March 1961, near Kano, and its construction had caused quite a commotion in the area. If our friend's description was correct, large sections of the station were trucked the 715 miles from the port at Lagos to the site.

As I went to get the movie screen from the storage closet, I pictured what it might be like if I lived my entire life deep in the bush and witnessed such a spectacle. I would have seen trucks before, and possibly trains. But nothing in my life's experience would have helped me make sense of this huge piece of NASA's station now moving toward my village—on the road I travel on foot or by oxcart or camel.

Even in the city, where planes flew in and out of Kano a few times a week, some people still couldn't make out what was inside those metal tubes and what kept them up in the sky. (Air traffic was still infrequent enough that each flight's arrival was heralded by the emir's trumpeter atop his camel, continuing the tradition that greeted the arrival of trans-Saharan camel caravans.)

A clinking sound and the aroma of coffee brought me back to the immediate preparations as Adamu carried a tray of cups from the kitchen. The men would be here any minute. I set up the screen. Adamu got out folding chairs, and he and I hurried to put out a few refreshments. Carl wrestled with the film, coaxing it through the Bell & Howell's threading mechanism.

His team members were English-speaking Nigerians, and some were graduates of the secondary school system. A few of them accepted that men had landed on the moon, or told Carl they did. I had to admit, it sounded impossible. And I mulled a question. When you struggle for mere survival, wouldn't it seem senseless to send men to walk around on the moon? Spending money that could have provided food, shelter and medical care to so many?

About a dozen men arrived in two SMP trucks, and Carl welcomed them into our home. Adamu served the refreshments. I faded into the background out of respect for a culture where women in most households remained hidden from men outside their immediate family. I gave a modest nod to the few who glanced in my direction.

After refreshments, the men settled into their seats, I sat down in a back corner and the whir of the projector called the group to order. A short history of flight and rocketry preceded details of lunar lander construction, astronaut selection and the rigorous tests of men and equipment.

Adamu joined the others in uproarious laughter at scenes of training for weightlessness. Views of the moonwalk were met with silence.

I observed the faces I could see from my corner. Expressions varied—amazed, suspicious, puzzled, amused. When the film ended, the men all left together with little conversation, and that only in Hausa.

"B-B, I think some of the guys were convinced. What do you think?" Carl was packing up the projector.

I said I wasn't sure. I thought a few showed a glimmer of acceptance that maybe, just maybe, the "fantasy" really happened.

Carl was silent for a moment, then looked at me over the top of his glasses. "So you think some of the guys were humoring me?"

Adamu smiled to himself as he picked up a tray of cups and left the room.

# 13

# EXPATS

*Expatriate.*

**Verb:** To banish or exile a person from his native country.

**Noun:** A person who lives outside his native country.

That's us. Expatriates, but entirely of our own choosing. Affectionately known as "expats," we venture far and wide, and can be found in all corners of the globe. Some spend entire careers as expats in one part of the world or another, either for years in one place or in a nomadic existence. The expat community worldwide is quite small, so we've encountered friends from another time and place, or friends of those friends, in the most remote outposts.

Kano introduced us to the expatriate life, a key ingredient of which is dinner partying in each other's homes. The scene is repeated wherever expats are found, and the stories exchanged become legends.

Since Muslim women would not have come to our home or invited us, we had no friendships with local couples. Our social life was with Indians, Brits and, of course, other Americans.

## Out of India

Expat Indian physicians and their families were a long-established presence in Kano and in the areas of British influence throughout the world. It was through them that I was introduced to Indian food.

Before living in Kano, my gustatory experience had been limited. Just a few short years before, friends in my small college town exchanged excited phone calls about the opening of a new café in town that served a one-dish meal called pizza. Now in Kano, in the homes of several Drs. Patel (a common name among Indian physicians), I dove into the riot of colors, aromas and flavors beckoning from long tables laden with seductive platters. Shimmering gold- or silver-embroidered saris accessorized the evenings. My senses did cartwheels.

Two doctors' wives taught me a few Indian cuisine basics. Lesson one, making ghee and grinding spices. (Fenugreek is hard to grind with a mortar and pestle, let me tell you.) Lesson two, minced lamb samosas, and lesson three, one of the many varieties of curry. I was hooked. Once we were back in the States, these dishes would constitute my go-to menu for dinner guests.

## Kano Club and the Brits

Descending from the ethereal heights of Indian cuisine, the old British Kano Club served up an uninspired but edible meal, the special Sunday lunch attracting the most patrons. Sunday, or any other day, our kids enjoyed eating something that went by the name "hamburger."

These venerable British clubs must be in every city throughout the former British Empire. Some say that the erstwhile colonials keep connected to home and to their feeling that the universe revolves around them by the nostalgia of the clubs and polo grounds, as well as BBC's *This Is London* and the sound of Big Ben tolling the hours of Greenwich Mean Time.

In Kano, the club was an unpretentious one-story structure. Low, white decorative block walls graced the main building, outdoor dining patio, and swimming pool area. Acacia and flame trees shaded the complex.

Carl and I read or socialized, shaded by thatch umbrellas at the tables around the pool. (Still no talk of the Nigeria-Biafra war.) Other adults swam or splashed about for a few minutes at a time to cool off. Charles and Ginger had near-exclusive possession of the kiddie pool since most English children were sent away to boarding school at age five.

With an independent Nigeria not quite ten years old, a large number of British civil servants and businessmen remained in the country. One of them shared a story in his best upper-crust accent about the old-timer whose watch had lost its minute hand. It didn't matter to the man, though, as he said, "I find that in Africa, one hand is quite sufficient." Our new acquaintance said to consider the African concept of time when having Africans over for dinner, but Malam Kazari had already initiated us to late arrivals and extra guests.

The Brits who had spent entire careers here enlivened our visits to the club. They regaled any willing listeners, of which we were certainly two, with vivid stories of adventure and adventurer, and tales of men who had been in Africa too long and had "gone bush."

Wood paneling imparted a warmth to the club's interior, and there was of course a portrait of Queen Elizabeth II. A dartboard in the pub drew enthusiastic adherents. If the Kano Club showed a film and newsreel from England, we all stood for "God Save the Queen."

Our attempt at golf came when Carl and I went with two other couples to the nine-hole course the Kano Club maintained. Persuading the donkeys and camels frequenting the course to yield right-of-way required time and patience.

## American Fun and Games

Besides our family and the USAID advisors from Ohio University, the American contingent in Kano consisted of a US Information Agency (USIA) officer, an agriculture advisor and a registered nurse, and their spouses. As I remember it, three of the Ohio families had young children with them in Kano.

The USIA officer was a polished and consummate communicator, as befitted his duties. He had previously served a tour somewhere in North Africa. So he introduced us to couscous and the most delectable meat specialties, served in style on his textile-adorned screened veranda.

The couple with the agricultural mission were pleasant, inviting and down to earth—no pun intended—and had been in Kano several years. They lived on the edge of town, next to the experimental farm, and enjoyed the shade and glorious blaze of color from the huge flame tree near their drive.

The nurse and her husband were congenital smilers. Both had the ability to laugh and look on the bright side of any circumstance. We weren't always glad to see Nurse Kathy because part of her job was to keep all of us up to date with our shots. But hers was the only table at which we confidently ate green salad. And somehow her bleach-soaked lettuce seemed fresher and crisper than mine.

The dozen Ohio families lived in a group of identical cube-like houses on wide yards on a one-block street. Sculptured shrubs relieved the visual monotony, but the shade and water under them attracted cobras. A couple of families, not just one, kept pet mongooses (not "mongeese") to combat the snake population. Our friends loved to recount the legendary accuracy of West African Spitting Cobras—how they can hit a victim's eye from eight feet or more, then kill with a bite. We took the lesson to heart—never make eye contact with a cobra. Besides the shrubbery and water trenches, these houses had a walled, covered garden patio attached to the house. Intended to provide a shaded area for relaxing and cooling off, such an area could no doubt attract prey for snakes, and therefore snakes, into the houses.

During daylight hours, we all had plenty to do, the men on their jobs and the wives managing the household, shopping in the markets or experiencing the culture. But at dusk, Kano rolled up the sidewalks, as they used to say in rural Oklahoma. Not to worry. The Ohio group invented diversions to keep us all entertained after the sun went down. A large cement slab in the middle of the block served many a purpose besides basketball or badminton. Twice a week the slab hosted square dances, presided over by the resonant voice of a big ruddy-faced extrovert, a professional caller. We went twice, and I found it great fun, but Carl didn't like it, so we didn't continue.

Once a month the slab became a theater. Folding chairs and a screen were set up for the movie sent to us on the US government circuit. We never received recent movies, and for a few months we concluded film studios had abandoned all movie-making except for spaghetti westerns. Africans walking by on the road, sometimes stopped to watch for a while. They laughed heartily at events we considered catastrophic. With the aforementioned spaghetti western genre, the rest of us enjoyed laugh therapy as well.

All-work-and-no-play Carl did make time for the movies and also listened to classical music on our record player when he could. (He often said he hoped to die listening to an opera at La Scala.)

Carl tended to make one close friend, or maybe two, in each place we lived. In Kano that friend was Tom Antorietto. They each had an unconventional way of looking at the world, and they bounced their bizarre sense of humor off each other to the great amusement of a few of us, especially themselves. Others within earshot could be heard to mutter under their breath, "huh?"

Carl regaled Tom and the rest of us with stories about his ideal places to visit and someday live—the most isolated destinations he could get to: The Outer Hebrides, the Azores, the island of St. Helena where the British had imprisoned Napoleon or Alice Springs in the middle of the Australian outback. Sounded way too isolated to suit me. And I hoped he'd never *actually* come in the door with those two tickets for the Trans-Siberian Railway from Moscow to Vladivostok.

We didn't join the Ohio bridge players and never witnessed those weekly sessions, but we heard tales. One group met at Tom's house and played the game for fun. But bridge as it was played at the science teacher's house wasn't for the faint of heart. Apparently, the fate of the free world hung precariously on the game's outcome.

Birthdays provided excuses for festive celebrations when no other excuse presented itself. Mine came soon after we arrived, and the Ohio friends made sure I didn't feel neglected. I received dubious proof I didn't look my thirty-two years when a twenty-something gal from the group said, "You are so *well preserved!*"

Then there was Halloween! Trick-or-treating to the dozen American houses was made as time-consuming and scary as each occupant's creativity could make it.

But something on Halloween night rattled the nerves of all the adults. One family returned home to find their tree hung with juju amulets—black magic. Obviously, someone had paid a witchdoctor to "witch" them. If the targeted family knew or suspected the reason for their being so targeted, it forever remained a mystery to the group.

Thanksgiving brought together all the Americans in Kano for a butter-infused feast. A donkey and donkey cart provided a hay-ride. Well, all right, there was no hay. But the eight children rode the donkey cart up and down the block as many times as they could negotiate.

My goodness! If that one-block street could tell tales . . .

One day, a woman who we were sure was American appeared in front of our house, just one in a crowd of people gathered in our yard. We were all intent on watching a parade that would end next door at Government House, home and offices of the military governor. The band paraded by on their camels, performing on their handmade instruments—horns of hammered metal, drums of animal hide stretched over a wood frame, and stringed instruments of animal hide and—well, string. I guessed the American stranger must be a professor of music or maybe an employee of a museum because she was intent on acquiring African musical instruments. I was itching to satisfy my curiosity about where this unknown person came from or how she had arrived in our yard in Kano. But she was focused on her mission. I didn't interrupt.

The woman thrust hands full of cash up to the musicians as they passed by. Some held out for better terms for a minute or two while she added more cash to her offer, but the men were all smiles by the end of their transactions. The parade's music became less robust with each of her purchases and was quite feeble by the time the procession arrived next door. Mission accomplished, the woman quickly disappeared into the crowd. We had never seen her before and never saw her again.

Carl met a group of US Peace Corps volunteers in the course of his work out in the villages and invited them to come in from the bush one evening and join us for dinner. Carl and I had con-sidered joining the Peace Corps several years earlier and enjoyed the evening's exchange with this group. A couple of women took the opportunity to have a hot bath before they left. But a few Peace Corpsmen appeared to look with disdain at the size and comfort of our house, as if living in the bush made their experience superior to ours.

I understood their attitude. After all, my childhood dream of life in Africa had me in a thatch-roofed hut far from civilization.

# 14

# PRIMA DONNA

*Charles turned five* not long after we arrived in Kano. Meninge arranged for camel rides, a popular birthday entertainment among the Americans. Camel and camel driver arrived before the cake and ice cream, and we all watched as the noble animal undulated up the road toward the house. Her blankets and red embroidered halter dripped with tassels, and the driver wore colored print daishiki and kufi.

The four-legged lady made her grand entrance into our dusty drive like a diva, regally turning her head in a rather disdainful survey of her adoring audience. I half expected her to pick up one padded foot and do the royal wave.

Up close, despite the surge of odiferous air, her cloven upper lip, doe-eyes, bushy eyebrows and long thick eyelashes won my enthusiastic, "Aww, what a swe-e-e-t face." That is, until she opened her mouth to broadcast a long, alien honk and expose her huge blotchy teeth. She stretched her long tongue around in the air with no apparent purpose. Bad breath front and center. Stage presence gone.

But the children had fun. They were as entertaining as the camel. While one rode, the other five little guests, just like the Pied Piper story, followed along in single file.

I was having fun watching them and taking pictures when the trouble began.

"C'mon, Bee. You should take a turn. You don't want to miss out."

The other American moms had done this before. Oh, all right. I guessed I'd be sorry later if I didn't try it.

The camel was resting, her favorite activity, belly on the ground, knees and legs folded under her. I used a step stool and climbed aboard, somehow managing it modestly, covered by the folds of my dress. The driver pointed out the handles on the front and back of the saddle. I extended my legs straight out in front, crossing them at the ankles. The camel ignored the driver's *rruuh!* command. Too busy chewing her cud. But then, with a sudden jolt, she obeyed.

"Ship of the Desert" took on new meaning—and me with no Dramamine. It all happened in far less time than it takes to tell. First, the camel rose to kneel on her front knees. I rolled up and backward a few degrees. Next, her back legs joined the upward trajectory. I pitched upward, forward and downward, the ground staring me in the face. Last, she straightened her front legs to a full stand. I rolled backward and up the vertical plane to arrive at my high-altitude destination. The driver waited for me to catch my breath, and then led Miss Doe-Eyes out of our driveway for a long, slow sashay up the road.

I was on trek across the Sahara. A bold explorer of that fabled desert.

But parts of my body, anchored in reality, registered relief when we came back around a bend and I once again sighted our driveway. After I lurched, pitched and rolled forward and back-ward again in the return to my mount's resting position, I stumbled off and tottered stiffly into the house.

"I think I'll just serve cake."

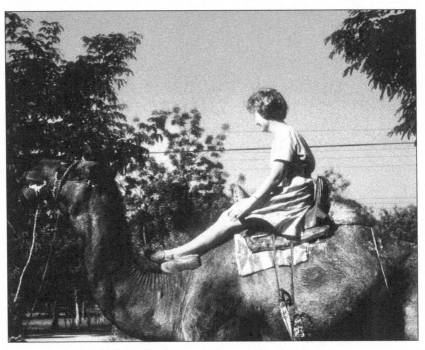

Bee ready for a trek across the Sahara

# 15

# HAUSA CUSTOMS

## Education

Here and there around Kano, we would see a white-robed
man sitting on the ground point to lines of Arabic on a wooden
board. Seven or eight young boys sat in a semicircle at his feet.
The man was an Islamic teacher, and the boys were learning to
recite the Koran.

We'd been given a helpful booklet, *Hausa Customs*. Three men
representing different (unspecified) regions of Hausaland com-
piled the book, and the Northern Nigerian Publishing Company
published it the year before we arrived. I often checked it for answers to my questions.

The only education information in the booklet, a section titled
"Islamic Studies," provided the following: After a boy has been
circumcised, at about age seven or eight, his parents give him a
pair of shorts, a shirt and a blanket and place him with a malam
for Islamic religious instruction. *Hausa Customs* says parents want
their sons and daughters to get Islamic religious instruction. The
authors go on to say, "It is this tradition which was responsible
for the strong opposition to Western education which was regarded as a clever way of indoctrinating the young children to the

Christian religion." (The authors used the past tense, thirty years before the founding of Boko Haram—words meaning "Western education is forbidden.")

In the eastern part of Hausaland, including Kano, emphasis is on memorizing the entire Koran. The passages are transcribed onto that wooden board I saw the malam using. After the entire book is learned completely by heart, the boy studies pronunciation and intonation.

In the western sector, emphasis is not on committing the entire Koran to memory, and after a certain point the reading is suspended and the study of Arabic grammar and literature begins. Then, after the boy can recite the first four sections of the Koran and read and transcribe the rest, he can move on to studying other subjects, such as math.

But in the booklet *Kano State,* published soon after we arrived, I learned that, in addition to Islamic schools, there were seven government secondary schools in the state, five for boys and two for girls. Of four teachers training colleges in the state, one was for women. These plus craft, technical and commercial schools and a branch of Ahmadu Bello University completed Kano State's educational opportunities.

## Marriage Customs

I looked up marriage in the booklet by the three Hausa authors.

Sections on the courtship, the bride price, the four wives permitted by Islam, and who arranges who marries whom fit with much of what I'd heard. But then I was in for a shock.

I read that child marriage is the rule rather than the exception in most parts of Hausaland. Many boys and girls are married off at the age of twelve or thirteen, and most boys in Hausaland are married before the age of twenty. When a husband is so young he can't even take care of himself, his parents have the responsibility for both.

*Hausa Customs* says one of the claims in favor of child marriage is that ". . . a girl comes to love and venerate her husband from a very early age and will become firmly attached to him as she grows up. As she has not reached the age of defiance (adolescence), a girl will readily accept her father's choice of a husband, which is all to the good because her father's choice is that of a wise and mature adult . . ."

The next section gave me chills.

In some rural parts of Hausaland, a girl is married away at the age of five or six. The girl actually goes to her "marriage home" at this age and is brought up by her husband, "but he doesn't have sexual relations with her until he thinks she is ready, certainly not before the age of twelve."

I thought of my eighteen-month-old daughter. Under this system, Carl could choose a man and marry Ginger off in three or four more years. I couldn't stand to think about it.

Then there was *forced marriage*, which *Hausa Customs* says is closely tied with child marriage: "Islam puts responsibility for a girl's marriage entirely on her father, if she has not attained the age of puberty. The father can give her away to a person of his choice without consultation with her or even her mother." The authors say this system is "capable of abuse," and some greedy fathers marry off their daughters to old men for "mercenary motives" or to someone close to royalty to gain prestige.

The high divorce rate in these situations has sullied the image of Hausa marriages, "both inside and outside the Hausa community." And when a father refuses to let his daughter divorce the husband he chose for her, she frequently runs away from home and becomes a prostitute.

In what pocket of my brain could I file all of this? I couldn't think of any positives in young children getting married, and the idea made me uncomfortable. Now if I saw a man and a little girl together in the market, I could no longer assume the pair was a father and daughter.

The authors say with the spread of Western education, child marriage and "its appendage, forced marriage," are disappearing from Hausa society. My Western brain was relieved.

But the booklet had one more surprise for me—Sadaka marriage. The father may, as an act of piety, give a daughter to a learned man or a poor man who cannot afford the usual financial arrangements. "The husband-to-be is not normally intimated of the event and his surprise when the bride is brought to his house can only be imagined." Some fathers do this in order to give away "an ugly daughter" rather than for pious reasons. If the girl is not pretty, a man may be bold and refuse, but respectfully and with regret, "because I do not have room enough in my house." The authors said this is what the man says even if he has four rooms (in other words, room for four wives) in his house. Sadaka marriage is also dying out.

## Some "Hausa Superstitions"

The *Hausa Customs* booklet's final chapter was "Some Superstitious Beliefs." Here is a sampling of the seventy-six listed by the authors.

1.  If a person sleeps in the same room as a leper, then he must never be the first to leave the room in the morning. If he does he will become a leper too. (The leprosy germs are believed to leave the body of the leper when he sleeps and congregate around the doorway.)

2.  If a small child is allowed to eat eggs, he will become a thief.

3.  Washing clothes on Wednesdays or Saturdays brings destitution, just as does (for a woman) plaiting the hair on Sundays or Wednesdays, or attending Koranic schools on Thursdays and Fridays, or spinning on Friday or Sunday nights by those whose mothers are still living.

4.  The person who finds money by the wayside must give half of it as alms to the poor, or else he will lose a lot more money than he originally found.

# 16

## FOR YOUR EYES ONLY

*While Carl was* at work, I wrote and posted a sister-to-sister confession:

> Dearest Peggy,
>
> This note is for your eyes only. I'll be quick. Sometimes I drive myself to Kingsway, the British grocery store. Driving on the left is challenge enough on the straightaway, but turning corners makes me a nervous wreck. The streets are jam-packed—thick with people and activity—and it would be so easy to hit a pedestrian or bicyclist. I'm sorry to tell you this is not a hypothetical statement.
>
> Last week I turned into what I thought was a clear lane. Out of nowhere a bicycle and its rider flipped up in the air and onto the hood of the truck. I was petrified. Had I injured the man, or worse? A dozen scenarios blitzed through my brain, none pretty. But the rider bounced off the hood as though it were a trampoline, gave me a brief matter-of-fact look, reunited body with bicycle and barreled on down the road. Few among the sea of pedestrians even glanced at the cyclist or at me, and those who did registered no surprise.

I thanked the Lord the situation wasn't far worse. First, I thought of all the horrible things I could have done to the cyclist. After I realized he appeared uninjured and had disappeared into the crowd, it hit me. Would there be consequences to me or to the US government? Yes, this was the truck with the US Agency for International Development shield and Smallpox Measles Program emblazoned on the side. There was no mistaking its identity. But the dozens of witnesses appeared to have no interest in me or in what had transpired. Body trembling, I pulled off the road as soon as possible. It took a while to calm myself enough to drive again.

I don't think I'll tell Carl.

# 17

# CRASH

*November 21, 1969:*

This is a sad day in our house. Yesterday's Nigeria Airways VC-10 flight from London to Lagos via Kano crashed into a teak forest on approach into Lagos. All eighty-seven people on board were killed. With so many passengers being from Kano, the mood in town is grim. Charles's British kindergarten teacher was among the dead. We'll talk to Charles, but I wonder how things will be when the students go back to school.

# 18

# TWO TARGETS

*All around us* there was death. Death from so many causes. But in Nigeria we were seeing the end of deaths from smallpox. Carl had a sense of accomplishment, and I was proud of him and his work. I couldn't imagine the reward felt by native vaccinators who made such a profound impact on the lives of their own families and neighbors. Smallpox had defied most efforts even to reduce its incidence. Now we were in this visionary campaign to conquer it once and for all.

And measles. Measles was a child killer. When Carl traveled in the bush, the sight of a whole cluster of fresh graves, all of them small, outside a village announced measles had recently swept through, taking the young children of the village with it. In West Africa, measles was not considered a good candidate for eradication. We would eradicate smallpox and control measles.

With these two killers in the crosshairs, CDC had determined the science supported attacking them simultaneously. The teams could give smallpox vaccine to everyone and measles vaccine to children between six months and three years (originally up to six years).

Carl was tenacious. Day after day, street by street, village by village, taking his meals from the village pot, he chased the two viruses. Chased them, isolated them, headed them off at the pass. Every operations officer, epidemiologist, vaccinator and driver did the same. From Mauritania to the Congo River, and from the Bight of Benin to the Sahara, the program moved with impressive speed. They overcame unimaginable problems and long delays. Heads of state, emirs and village chiefs put out directives or enticements supporting vaccination. Sometimes they acted out of fear of the disease, and sometimes out of their own self-interest to enhance their image and position. Regardless, it all happened faster than anyone had thought possible.

And the surveillance-containment method, which was renamed Eradication-Escalation, surprised most with the speed with which it reduced outbreaks. CDC had hired people who, besides being flexible enough to manage two different methods at the same time, had proven themselves to be expert as disease detectives to discover where the virus had come from and where it was likely to go next. Carl and others took the find-and-contain approach and ran with it. The West and Central Africa Smallpox Eradication Program headed into the home stretch.

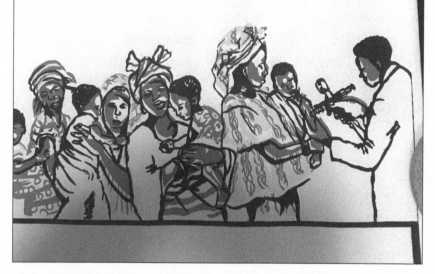

Hausa language smallpox-measles vaccination poster

# 19

# HEMORRHAGIC FEVER

*A startling discovery* was made not far from Kano State in 1969:

There's been quite a stir around here lately—a new hemorrhagic fever discovered and spreading in Borno State. Two nuns who worked in a mission in the village of Lassa died earlier this year of a mysterious disease that causes tiny hemorrhages all over the body. Researchers at Yale finally identified the virus and have named the disease "Lassa fever." It's carried by a type of rat whose choice abode is people's houses, where it sheds the virus in its urine and feces. (I'd better show pictures to Adamu and Audu so they can help me be on the alert.) Eating the rats puts a person at even greater risk than any other type of contact, but in some quarters this rat is a delicacy!

We don't know how contagious it is yet, but people are kind of sweating it because of the new book, *Andromeda Strain*. The man who led the research and discovered the virus got sick from it back in the summer and nearly died. Yale shut down the research on the virus after a lab worker died. The smallpox operations officer over in Maiduguri, and the one down in Jos, have been cabled (it's not like you can just pick up a phone) to drop everything and go help with the disease detective work. I guess they'll leave smallpox duties in the hands of their teams. I'm crossing my fingers Carl doesn't have to go.

# 20

## JUST WHO CARL WAS

*Why was it* my husband could not say no when the need was greatest? He would have left in a flash to help with the Lassa fever epidemic, or in the Ebola crisis if that disease had been around at the time.

Fortunately for me and our children, it turned out CDC had enough teams who were closer to Lassa and Borno State. Carl wasn't needed. But he would have gone. That's just who Carl was. He had a passion for coming to the rescue of difficult causes, hopeless causes, people in distress. He had such a concern for others and made them feel so cared for that few knew he often had to go off by himself to recharge his batteries. (My father could hardly stand to be away from my mother, so it had taken me a few years to realize that this need of Carl's didn't mean a lack of love for me.)

Carl's kind of love would be demonstrated in a very poignant way a decade into the future in Saudi Arabia. He became aware of a young man, Hisham, whose dune buggy accident had broken his neck and left him a quadriplegic but who had taught himself to draw using a pencil held in his mouth. Carl created a contract to bring Hisham in a couple of days a week to work on the health education graphics team. On the first morning, Carl asked his driver to go to the village where Hisham lived and bring him to the office. Alawi refused Carl's request even though he adored Carl and our entire family. Then two other staffers refused the task. When Carl called a meeting to get to the bottom of the issue, he learned that his local staff believed God wanted Hisham to stay hidden, or the injury would not have happened. They believed they would be thwarting the will of God if they brought Hisham to work.

So Carl drove to the village himself each time, physically picked Hisham up and carried him to the car, then carried him in from the car when he arrived back at his offices. One of Carl's nursing staff later told him that the clerk, on watching this scene one day, remarked, "Mr. Bloeser has an angel in him."

# 21

## MEDIEVAL FESTIVAL

*Day 1—morning:* The festival of Eid al Fitr had arrived. It marked the end of Ramadan, a month of official fasting from dawn till dusk and unofficial eating and partying from dusk till dawn. (The delicious aromas wafting from Adamu's quarters during Ramadan could wake us from a sound sleep during the night.) But now Eid was here. The mood was electric.

One of the emir's wives, the third wife to the best of my memory, had a special relationship with a couple of Ohio University wives—not surprising given her husband's advocacy for improved education. This charming lady, whom I will refer to as the princess, invited us to the women's courtyard to witness the ceremonial return of the emir's procession after it opened the festival at the vast prayer grounds.

We passed through a set of interior gates in the mud walls of the medieval palace and entered the courtyard of the harem. Except when an emir permitted it for special occasions, no one could enter this courtyard but women, children and eunuchs. The harem may not be what you imagine. The word simply means the wives and concubines of a polygamous man. We did not see dancing girls with jeweled navels. There were no diaphanous veils, no satin pillows, no servants with palm fronds fanning the ladies or dropping grapes into their mouths.

After we watched the royal procession parade through the courtyard (more about this later), the princess invited us to return in the late afternoon for drumming and dancing. We were happy to accept.

Day 1—evening: We American wives arrived to find thirty or more women—wives, concubines, servants—and their children in a half circle already pulsating. The drummers' hands were a blur. And the drums! A huge calabash gourd turned upside down floated on water in yet a larger gourd. Various sizes of drums created tones from deep, round and rich to high and thin. Other drums consisted of animal hides stretched over a bowl-shaped wood framework or hides stretched over the end of a hollowed-out log.

The music throbbed and energized the group. The women shuffled and swayed with their heads down, eyes on their feet, gracefully weaving the colors of wrappers and turbans into a moving tapestry. A young boy danced in the center. He leapt and crouched and whirled—whirled so fast! Would he vaporize right out of sight? The women urged him on, clapping, pumping the air with their fists and cheering him with the high-pitched trilling sound. Then they began to urge us—the three Americans—to take center stage, and two of us finally gave in, doffing our shoes and kicking up the dust to their cheers. I had captured the boy's feverish performance on film but was grateful no one picked up my camera to film me.

Day 3: The crowning event was the Kano Durbar. The emir would make his pageant-filled entry onto the palace square and take his place at the main gate. People from all the chiefdoms in his realm would pay their respects. Carl and I arrived early to look for the best place to stand. We hoped for shade. But the double row of neem trees lining the drive to the main gate provided the only relief from the sun on the square's acres of dirt. Carl pointed to a spot near the gate. "Let's just get a good vantage point—forget fighting for a sliver of shade."

In future years the Kano Durbar would expand and become a major tourist attraction. But in 1969 we were but a handful of expatriates. In the harem I'd had a taste of the processional Carl and I would see today. For us as Christians, this was not a religious festival, but we could watch and enjoy the pageantry.

Over the next hour, thousands of people streamed into the square. Bodies jostled, merging sweat with unidentified perfumes and oils. Aromas jousted with odors, which competed with the buzz of voices, horns and bells, which in turn fought to upstage visual display.

In contrast to the men's everyday white and pale blue shirts and tunics, brash prints showed off intense colors. The designs dipped and soared through saffron orange, bright yellows, flame tree red, blues and greens. The same colors swathed women in their two-meter-long wrappers, matching blouses and swirled turbans. The sight was all the more dramatic as the colors framed obsidian skin.

Suddenly, noise levels soared. Chiefs and their equestrian groups were arriving, reining in their high-spirited desert steeds. Hooves pawed the earth. I wound the 8mm. Each chiefdom's group of horses and riders wore matching attire. Bold colors, gold and silver embroidery surging in, around and over the colors, saturated the vestments and silk turbans. The sun glinted off chain mail or pieces of recycled tin, with designs hand cut or hammered and made into ornamental suits of armor. Full battle array. The horsemen brandished ceremonial swords. As the start time drew nearer, the horsemen moved to the far edge of the expanse fronting the palace. Near us, beads of sweat glistened on faces in the afternoon sun, but no one seemed to mind the wait. Time didn't matter.

Then someone spotted the lead riders off in the distance. The crowd's animation escalated. Tinkling miniature bells and jangling handmade metal ornaments on the tack of horse and camel grew louder as they approached. The procession passed within ten or fifteen feet of Carl and me, almost as close as when I was in the harem courtyard. The camel-mounted musicians produced haunting desert music on their native drums and horns, lutes and lyres. The elaborate embroidery and the visual and auditory display so overwhelmed me, I don't remember noticing the smells that accompany a horse and camel parade.

Emir Ado Bayero, seated on a throne-like perch atop his mount, wore white robes and the royal headdress—a white turban tied at the top, forming two rabbit ears. A courtier twirled the royal white-and-pale-blue tasseled umbrella above him. Flanked by his guards, he took his place in front of the palace gate not more than twenty yards from where we stood. The trumpeters raised their *kakaki*, twelve-foot-long medieval ceremonial trumpets. Across the square, the riders maneuvered their horses into position.

Then the blast from the trumpets.

The first team of riders bolted like lightning across the square, churned up the dusty ground, pulled up—abrupt, vertical—rearing their horses inches in front of the emir. They extended an arm in salute, and then turned off to the side as the next group moved into position.

Charge—lightning speed—thundering hooves—clouds of dust—salute—cheers! One team moved to the side, and we caught our breath before the next.

Carl shouted above the roar, "Must be a movie camera hidden somewhere."

"Yeah. Cast of thousands. The director will yell, 'Cut!' any minute now!"

"What?!"

"Cast of thousands!!"

The next group moved into position.

Charge—lightning speed—thundering hooves—clouds of dust—salute—cheers!

It was like a rodeo and a horse race rolled into one.

During each lull in the action, I caught my breath and got our camera ready. Just when I thought the crowd's excitement could go no higher, it climbed again with the next climactic salute. In wave after wave of horsemen, each chiefdom strove to outdo the one before it. High-octane energy. Hooves thundered. High-pitched, throaty trilling piercing the air merged with the thunder pounding in my head.

As the last team of horsemen paid homage, a deafening roar ended the ceremony. I tried to clear dust from my eyes and nose. The Durbar itself had lasted less than an hour, perhaps as little as half an hour. As the sun sank low enough to cast shadowy fingers, the emir and his entourage passed through the gate into the palace.

# 22

# WINDS OF SAHARA

*Christmas of 1969* came before I knew it, and it was time to update family and friends with a year-end newsletter.

I wish you could see our crystal-clear night sky. With no streetlights, we've had nights with darkness so profound you'd think handfuls of diamonds had been thrown out across black velvet.

But we won't see a sky like that for a while now. Harmattan has arrived. I'd never heard of it, but now I'll never forget it. It's the season of Saharan winds, although I'd call them breezes, that for several weeks each year carry part of the Sahara to all points south, and even across oceans. We hear about years when planes can't land and when you "can't see your hand in front of your face." Clouds of grit and flour-like dust invade every crevice. The grayish-beige sky tends more toward gray as charcoal heaters outside homes add smoke and toxins to the mix. (Many insulate their huts with animal dung, so add odors to the above.) I try to shield my eyes, nose and lungs, and I brush flecks of soot off my clothes. But we welcome the blessed relief from the heat.

I'm using the time to study the journals I brought with me. (By the way, as a fledgling speech pathologist, I'd love to examine some mouths around here. The *Hausa Customs* booklet tells about a baby's naming ceremony, seven days after its birth. One of the day's events is the barber shaving the baby's head, making any tribal markings requested by the father, and "removing the uvula"! I can't believe I haven't heard a lot of nasal-sounding voices!)

A quiet Christmas is on the horizon. The local people, being Muslim, don't celebrate Christmas, and we haven't found other Christians here to worship and be in fellowship with. Most other Americans and the Brits will go on leave. One couple we were with in Atlanta, stationed about five hours south of here in Jos, may take a break from the Lassa fever epidemic and drive up to visit for a couple of days. I'd prefer to go there instead. East Africa has highlands and many areas with a mild climate. In West Africa the Jos plateau is the only place that's similar. I've heard it's really pretty, not to mention cool. At many other smallpox posts, our colleagues live near a beach or a river. I've heard one of the wives swims in the same watering hole as hippos. Last thing I'd want to do.

I went out in our yard and got a spindly little bush that looks more like a New Mexico tumbleweed than a tree. But we'll make it festive. Charles is making a construction paper chain, aluminum foil balls, and popcorn garlands, and Ginger is trying to help. No nativity set or lights for the tree, but our emergency stash of candles for the frequent power outages will be Christmassy distributed around the room, and *The Night Before Christmas* made it into our air shipment.

Carl will of course ham it up with his operatic baritone

renditions. I do so wish I could harmonize with him without throwing him completely off. Solo, he can sing beautifully but always clowns around with it.

I'll make my usual fudge. Daddy, I'll try your divinity recipe, but it'll take years of practice and a stronger right arm to match your expertise at whipping up those perfect satiny peaks. Do people at church still call you the Doctor of Divinity?

When I put in our commissary order last month, I requested pecans, extra sugar, and canned sweet potatoes, green beans, and cranberry sauce. I ordered a tin of cocoa so we can have hot chocolate on Christmas Eve, and I'll try the recipe from the Women's Club cookbook for making my own marshmallows. The commissary order should arrive tomorrow in plenty of time to prepare.

We'll buy an extra-large hen from the bicycle vendor at the front door and pretend it's a turkey.

I hope all of you have a wonderful Christmas. We'll really miss being with you.

Much love to all and a very merry Christmas,
Bee and family

# 23

## MAKING VINEGAR

*A sampling from* the Kaduna International Women's Club Cookbook and Kitchen Guide

*Pineapple Vinegar:*

Cut ripe pineapple, including rind, to fill an enamel pail.
Cover with rain water or filtered water and a cloth.
Set in the sun for 3 weeks.
Strain, boil the liquid 30 minutes.
Put in sterile bottles.

*Cottage Cheese:*

Boil 2 C milk (Use prepared powdered milk if no fresh milk available.)

When it reaches boil, add mixture of 2 tsp vinegar and 2 tsp water.

Stir well and remove from heat.

In a few minutes it's ready to strain through a cheese cloth.

Add a bit of salt, and add a bit of milk if you want it richer. Cool immediately.

Fighting cooking odors: (from Mrs. G. of Pakistan)

When deep-frying anything, hang a damp cloth near to the pot to absorb odor.

When cooking fish, sprinkle cinnamon on the stove, or in the oven if baking.

*Weevils in flour:*

(Critters with varying numbers of legs love whole grains. We say that in Africa we can't count grams of protein in our food because of all the extra protein crawling in it.)

If you prefer not to eat them, try the following:

If too many to sift out, put in low oven, then sift.

If so many they create an odor, you can still use it to make bread for the dog.

*A few pidgin-to-English terms:*

Chop = food, a meal
Small chop = a snack
I wan chop = I want to eat
Small-small = a very small amount
It's finish = they ran out
Were you dey? = Where are you?

*Banish mosquito bite itch:*

Keep a one-gallon jar on your kitchen cabinet.

Fill with water and 1 to 2 tablespoons natural, e.g., Adolph's, meat tenderizer, dissolved.

After being bitten by mosquitoes, splash the above mixture liberally on all affected areas.

(The active ingredient, papain, draws the toxin out of the bite.)

# 24

# THE WAR ENDED TODAY

*Journal note—Thursday night,* January 15, 1970

The civil war ended today. Biafra surrendered. But what a strange day. Up here in the north, just as there's been no sense the country was in a civil war, today caused barely a blip on the radar. No doubt some Hausa families suffered a loss or waited at home for the return of a son or brother, but none I knew of. From our house, we heard no horns blaring or throngs in the streets when it was announced the war was over. I know people must be celebrating in Lagos and in areas near the war zone. With no telephone or radio and with news taking weeks to arrive, we could have a long wait for details of the surrender. The Ohio people should get some word over their shortwave radio. Adamu and Audu didn't say much, but they had big smiles when we said we heard the war was over.

———

## Things we learned later

The Nigerian president, Gen. Yakabu "Jack" Gowon, a moderate man who was well respected by the Americans, refused to have war crimes trials. "No victor, no vanquished," he said. He pardoned everyone, promoted reconciliation. We would learn he sought to model himself after Abraham Lincoln. On his visit to Kano some weeks after the war ended, I got a picture of him standing in his open-top car during his parade to Government House. He was highly praised in Kano State even though he was not a northerner and was a Christian.

After leaving the country, we would hear grumbling about an American ambassador in Lagos—Matthews, I think his name was—and his stance during the war. Our foreign service officers in Cameroon complained they'd had a hard time getting good information out of Lagos because the ambassador was too pro-federalist. Not his role, they said. His job was to communicate between his own country and the host country, not to take sides in their internal affairs. And then there were all the ways Cold War politics played into the war, even though the US was officially neutral.

I had so much to learn.

# 25

# PARTY IN THE HAREM

*Two American friends* and I with our four children in tow carted presents, balloons, a Coleman jug of Kool-Aid, and a birthday cake through the palace gate. The date was February 2, 1970. The emir's son, Nasiru, turned six years old that day.

We knew our way. Passing through a couple of outer gates, we soon entered the harem's familiar courtyard. Our children kicked their sandals into the dust as we headed across the mud-walled courtyard where a couple of us had kicked up some dust ourselves—back during the big festival. An ancient tree's gnarled trunk provided the one spot of interest in the long colorless rect-angle.

We said happy birthday to Nasiru. He returned a shy smile. His mother, the princess, greeted us with her usual warmth and grinned at the sight of the cake and balloons. For Nasiru's birth-day, the princess wore a beautiful purplish wrapper embossed with gold. The shimmer of a purple silk turban framed her face. She was lovely.

The brightly painted room where the princess received us on our visits was sparsely furnished. In my memory, the room was about fifteen feet square. The ceiling, at least twelve feet high, was painted with geometric designs and curved lines, and I captured its deep green, crimson and gold colors with my camera. Several wooden chairs lined the wall to our left as we entered.

The bed, also in this room, stood in an alcove a step up from the rest of the room. Its elaborately carved wood frame and its four posts held the foundation and mattress high off the floor. I would have needed a stepladder to climb onto that bed. I don't remember much about the fabric in the canopy, just that I loved the rich colors and the Eastern, maybe Persian, design.

The princess had been educated in England before her marriage, but as a wife of an emir she was now secluded within palace walls. She seemed to relish our visits. In her refined British English, she asked about our children and our parents, and talked about Nasiru and current events and fashion trends in England and America. Nurse Kathy brought her an American fashion magazine or two on each visit.

A few weeks earlier, the princess had invited these two Ohio women and me to come for lunch in her private quarters. Her tiny table-for-two managed to accommodate the three guests. We sat snug and squeezed between the walls of her kitchenette. (Based on other recounted lives in similar households, I'm sure she did little cooking and took most meals in a communal setting with a group of other women in the family.) She served us coarse bread and the groundnut soup common to the sub-Saharan area. Peanuts, or groundnuts, were a major cash crop and often provided the protein in the diet. When Americans or Europeans make this stew, we add lamb, chicken or beef, but when I was served it in Nigeria, it consisted of ground peanuts, broth and spices.

On Nasiru's birthday, after our usual exchange of pleasantries, we got right down to the business at hand. We put six candles on the cake. We arranged presents, the cake, and cups of Kool-Aid on a table that had been set up in the sitting room/bedroom. Everyone helped blow up the balloons—part of the fun—and we hung crepe paper garlands around the table. We introduced Nasiru to the game of pin-the-tail-on-the—uh, camel. Then we went through the ritual: open presents, light candles, sing "Happy Birthday," blow out candles, serve cake. Charles and one other American boy were close to Nasiru's age. They played nicely together, and the young prince took a gentle big-brother attitude toward Ginger. We Americans had fun, and the princess and her son seemed to enjoy the novelty.

"And now, I have a surprise for you," she said, and led us out her door. We were familiar with a fraction of this multi-acre complex, which we were told even included an Islamic school for the palace children and living quarters for hundreds of occupants. A small city. The princess and an escort led us through other walled passageways into a palace garden for a visit with the emir. Seated in a garden, not a throne room, and without the royal headdress, he didn't look like he'd be the object of those galloping high-speed salutes at Durbar. He thanked us for honoring Nasiru and chatted with us and our children. He expressed his appreciation for the work my companions were doing with the Teachers College and for Carl's work to eradicate smallpox.

———

The man we met that February day in 1970, Emir Ado Bayero, the thirteenth Fulani emir of Kano, was said to be one of the most cosmopolitan in Nigeria. He believed education was Nigeria's door to progress. He expanded colleges—Ado Bayero University in Kano is named after him—and he advocated for women's education, earning both praise and condemnation.

In 2020 Nasiru became emir of Bichi. But seven years prior, he was seriously injured along with his father and one of his brothers when gunmen attacked their convoy, killing a bodyguard and driver. The attack came near the end of his father's life and fif-ty-one-year reign and was widely believed to be a Boko Haram attempt to assassinate the emir. In one conflicting view, unknown persons have claimed in the Nigerian press that Nasiru was the actual target. They claim the attack was perpetrated by a purist Fulani faction bent on preventing Nasiru succeeding his father as emir because his mother was Yoruba.

But on that day in the palace, we simply enjoyed an innocent six-year-old boy's birthday.

# 26

# MARKET WITH A PAST

*Stateside shopping was* going to seem dull after living in Africa. Food vendors ringing their bicycle bells at our front door, the central market and the British grocery store all introduced me to a new sensory cornucopia. But American friends had promised the Kurmi Market in Kano's Old City would do that and more. I simply must see it. So when Carl had one of his rare office days and Meninge was available to drive us, Charles, Ginger, Adamu and I piled into the truck.

About twenty minutes from the house, we drove through one of thirteen gates in the Old City's eleven-mile mud wall on which construction began around AD 1200. In 1903 a British expeditionary force conquered Kano when they found the weak link, a flimsy gate. It is reported that at the time the wall was an unbelievable hundred feet thick at the base and as much as fifty feet high. Some sources say it even had moats, protected lookouts for sentries and terraces for horsemen to gallop around, protected by a continuous battlement.

Since then, the wall has been pilfered for building material and pounded down by the few torrential rains, and in many places is now only a mound of dirt ten or twenty feet high. But sections of the wall that frame the principal gates still soar upward and command respect.

Kurmi Market began in infamy, established over five hundred years ago as a slave market. Grim reports were that the city wall was fortified to protect the large amount of human property the Hausa had captured in their raids on weaker neighboring tribes to the south.

For centuries, Kano was a southern terminus of the trans-Saharan trade routes. Before Portuguese seafarers opened alternative avenues between sub-Saharan Africa and the north, caravans carried rock salt to West Africa, and pepper, spices and gold back to the north. That is, until the northbound traders found trade in human beings more lucrative. Caravans averaged one thousand camels, and on occasion many times that, fattened for the journey. On our first market visit, I was blissfully ignorant of its ignoble past and could enjoy the cultural experience.

Meninge parked the truck. I grabbed our bottles of purified water and my string bag, a net that would fit in a pocket and stretch to become a large sack. On the market's outer edge, we passed an open lot, a parking place for camels. Except for the constant chewing, they rested and waited for their next cargo, or next owner. I looked around for a Hertz Rent-a-Camel sign, or signs claiming "low miles—only one owner!"

Within the main Kurmi market, we came first to a wide sunny expanse where men worked with handsaws, hammers and nails, making furniture. The lumber from the forested south would crack as it dried in the Sahel's climate. Did they build the furniture out in the sun to hasten the drying before finishing the product? I spied twins and cousins of our sofa in various stages of construction.

Still out in the open area, our next stop was at a concrete slab, raised to allow blood to run off into the dust. But at this meat market most of the meat had yet to be liberated from the carcasses of old cows, hanging and dripping blood. I knew from our central market days Adamu knew which slab of meat, hacked at random from the carcass, could be made more tender for "European." He said something in Hausa, pointed to an area on the side of a carcass, and the butcher swung his machete. And as always, Adamu had advice. "Madame, this meat good. We can make soft." We put the bloody chunk in the string bag and would give it a good dose of meat tenderizer when we got home.

Battalions of flies blanketed any precut chunks of meat and organs laid out in the sun. I passed on that. Passed on quickly, away from meat spoiling or on the verge.

Next was leather work. Makes sense, I guess: meat—hides. Kano leather, a principal export, had made a name for itself. Kano's red goat hides are known as *Moroccan leather*. Donkeys carried loads of dried hides, like giant stiff flakes, from the countryside. The next step was tanning and softening, with the aid of cow urine.

Skilled craftsmen finished leather into handbags, bridles and camel saddles. After watching them work, I purchased two supple black leather hassocks, with a geometric design in the center made from the skin of a puff adder. These would make it to our living room floor after we aired them out in the sun for several days to dissipate residual odors, and then stuffed them with wads of paper.

We reached the crowded maze of stalls. Bamboo partitions separated them, thatch or corrugated metal shaded them and a mix of incense and other aromas filled the air. The noise of haggling escalated.

Adamu was on the job again. "Madame, we not buy with this man. Too much talk. Palaver. Plenty palaver."

From another vendor's dusty wooden shelves, Adamu chose a galvanized tin pail and a large painted enamel basin with a bold geometric design to take home to his wife—geometric because Islam forbids representations of people or animals.

Charles watched the artisans who lined these uneven dusty paths. He liked the potters and calabash carvers from nearby villages. Some men did intricate needlework on robes and kufis. I bought an ostrich feather fan and a basket. Adamu bought a horsehair fly whisk.

Any time Adamu and I shopped at the central market, it was much more crowded than this, and Adamu had to press our way through the sea of men. No other white people were in the Kurmi market today, but several buyers and sellers were women. They wore their native wrappers, sometimes combined with a knit shirt, sometimes not. I wore a respectful loose-fitting dress with modest neckline and sleeves.

Long unfamiliar somethings hung from a post to our right— kind of a stiff spongy-looking web of fibers. Meninge said they're loofahs, the "bushman's bath sponge."

Ginger's short legs tired, and it was hot. To my relief, Meninge offered to carry her.

Crocodile and cheetah handbags that traders brought from other parts of Africa occupied an artful display at the stall of a smartly dressed vendor. I bought crocodile handbags for Mother and my sister and one for myself. And, much as I hate to admit it now, I bought a cheetah handbag for an aunt.

Ahead of us, a crowd of children shouted, clamored and jumped around, trying to see over and around each other. What had them so excited? Was a handler showing off his mongoose fighting a cobra? No, it was a display of toys made of cheap plastic. The bright-colored novelties must have looked more fun than their hand-whittled toys. Charles spent his allowance on a toy rocket ship, and Meninge bought a hollow green plastic doll for Ginger.

At the food stalls I bought unidentified greens. Adamu, as usual, bought bottles of soda pop. I was surprised when he bought chew sticks (sugar cane stalks) and a few coveted caffeine-rich ko-lanuts. Men sit in front of their houses, chewing on a chew stick or on the kolanuts that stain their teeth but give them energy. The nuts are given as gifts during certain ceremonies. Adamu must have enjoyed these diversions in private because I'd never seen him chewing them. Of course, I'd never seen Adamu just sitting either.

The Hausa had a reputation as astute traders and business-men. They had a long history of trade with southern Yorubaland and with Lagos, since before Europeans arrived. Although many items were traded in each direction, we were told, as the 1970s approached, the main item drawing the Hausa traders that far south was the kolanut.

Kurmi Market would one day become popular with Ameri-can, British and Asian tourists for its African artifacts, and gov-ernments would ask UNESCO to name it a World Heritage Site. But that day was years in the future as this solitary foreigner drank in the experience.

The breezes of harmattan, with the few weeks of relief from the heat, had come and gone. Temperatures soared again as we approached the end of February. Clouds of flies swarmed around piles of garbage. They landed on beggars' sores and grimy tattered tunics, and on lips and eyes of animals and people. Evaporation in the dry air kept me, and my dress, from dripping perspiration, but I was hot and tired.

Open sewers, which we carefully stepped over all day, re-minded me we needed bleach baths for our produce. With the Sahara radiating heat like a solar furnace, the odor finally passed my tolerance level, and I was ready to return to the house and recline under the ceiling fan.

We cautiously reboarded our truck, its door handles and seats baked to well done. As Meninge pulled away from the market and onto the street, he pointed out the thick black stripe on top of a huge metal building. Buzzards! Shoulder to shoulder on the roof spine of the slaughterhouse, the feathered clean-up crew stood ready for its shift. The buzzards would take over and do their usual thorough job as soon as humans left the market. They approach their job with such passion. I was sorry we'd have to do without this dedicated crew in city life back in the States.

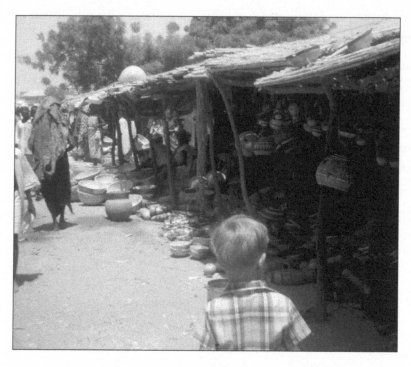

In Kurmi Market, Kano, Nigeria, 1969

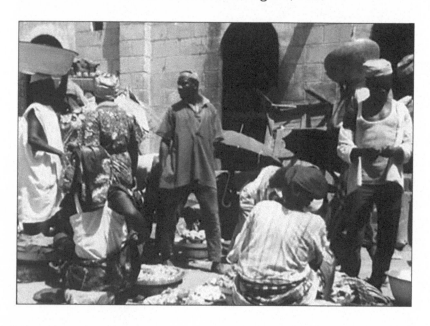

# 27

# OBJET D'ART

*Artful displays of* brass, wooden tribal masks and figures, thorn carvings and strands of African trade beads appeared at our door each evening as the succession of traders began about six o'clock. Each trader laid out a mat and arranged his items to show them in their best light before he rang the bicycle bell to announce his arrival. At least three or four traders, not always the same ones, came at various times throughout the evening.

They had learned for "Europeans" the rule was "the older the better." I watched for signs that indicated a recent carving or piece of brass had been buried in the dirt, thrashed with chains, or abused in some other way to "age" the item to antique status. Their favorite pitch line—"old-old, madame."

When seeking genuine local art, expats favored Sarki Trader and his shop for masks, drums, stools and carved figures. Sarki (Chief) specialized in old-old items he swore were authentic. To visit him, we navigated the treachery of uneven and potholed walking paths and crossed the rickety wooden planks spanning open sewers. (When we drove around town with our nostrils safe inside the Dodge, the stench didn't matter. This was different.) In the shop's cooler interior, we sat on carved African stools, drank cups of strong tea, fanned ourselves with ostrich feathers and took our time choosing from among the hundreds of objet d'art, the most intriguing ones draped with the cowry shells, historically used as currency. All were at a "special price just for you, madame."

One of the most ubiquitous items our front door vendors, and even Sarki, displayed were necklaces of African trade beads. The beads didn't appeal to me at the time, but most expats liked them. One of our program managers from CDC, a Princeton man through and through, wanted me to take him to Sarki Trader to buy African art every time he made the trip from Atlanta. Each time, he bought armfuls of trade bead necklaces. Just before we left Kano, I gave in. *Well, I guess I should buy at least one.* I remember I paid fifty cents.

After our return to the US, I would one day walk through Neiman Marcus out of curiosity. The higher the floor, the higher the price. On about the fourth floor, a jewelry island of locked glass cases sat in the center of all the racks of designer dresses. I was shocked to spot in the case a necklace of trade beads. Granted, they were of higher quality than those in my fifty-cent item. When I asked the price, the saleslady rather imperiously responded, "Madame, these are African trader beads. This piece is $285."

In my earliest days in Kano, I fell victim to the tag-team gambit at our front door. The first vendor spread out his wares in a way that showcased a single brass mortar and pestle, gleaming among all the other items. He didn't pitch it. He just waited for me to notice and comment on it, and even then didn't appear eager to sell it. We bargained. I don't remember how much I paid. I just know it was too much.

Moments later a different vendor came, saw my mortar and pestle that I had proudly displayed, and expressed a great desire to buy it from me for much more than I had paid. Wow! Wasn't I clever? I had obviously out-negotiated the first vendor if this item was worth so much. No, I was absolutely not going to sell it! Now it was time for the last member of the team, The Closer, I presume. From him I purchased four more, at a higher price than I had paid for the first one. At the end of our Africa tour, each relative received a brass mortar and pestle for Christmas.

## Reflection

sunset's stage presence
in dusty Sahel
mysterious, complex

plays roles bold or coy
commanding or supportive

flat-topped acacia tree
silhouette cliché
perfect sphere
dives
down

dare not look away

orb slips pale-gold body
into robe of rust-colored gauze
sheer lavender scrim
materializes onstage

behind it
golden circle inches toward purple exit
reaches down
touches darkening horizon of sand and ochre clay

soft and gentle
pulls the curtain behind it
slowly, then quickly, slips from sight

takes the day
all the day
along with it

in barely five minutes
theater is dark
the dark profound

# 28

# WOMEN HIDDEN
# BEHIND WALLS

*Four women in* colorful turbans and wrappers and carrying clip-
boards led me through a vaulted narrow gate in the wall that tow-
ered over us. Once inside Kano's Old City, we ducked through an
opening in another mud wall and emerged into a maze of walls
separated by narrow paths. We had a job to do over the next three
days.

With mass vaccination in Nigeria completed, the focus now
was on assessment and surveillance for quick containment of any
new smallpox outbreak. In such a survey of a population, the
percentage of people without scars of either the vaccination or
the disease itself would indicate whether a statistically significant
"pool of susceptibles" existed. If such a pool were present, Carl
would have to quickly mobilize all program resources.

But there was a problem. Carl and the men on his teams were
forbidden to go behind these walls. Most women living here were
in *purdah*, not to be seen by any man outside their own family.
My four health department guides had completed the assessment
in the Old City, but they had reported data the epidemiologists
knew could not possibly be correct. The job had to be repeated,
and soon. Carl needed corrected data for the upcoming visit of

the EIS officer. He trained me to assist in gathering the crucial statistics, and I relished the opportunity to see a life hidden from outsiders.

The SMP's surveillance protocol identified our start point on the map, and we proceeded from there in a direction and pattern dictated by a statistical grid. In rigid compliance with the pattern, we checked for the tell-tale scars and recorded our results.

The women on our team were reserved, at least with me, a foreigner there to help them redo their job. I followed their lead and reined in my usual talkativeness. The women spoke in Hausa to each other, and the team leader interpreted for me. I smiled a lot.

Mud formed everything within the Old City—walls, ovens, fire pits, houses. The twisting paths separating mud walls were narrow but not crowded with people since women in *purdah* were confined to their own compound. Few men were visible anywhere. (I was told that men spent their days in modern Kano shopping, working and socializing.) Even so, the tight passage could be tortuous, as human excrement, a black tributary to the larger open sewer, made its uneven way down the middle of the path.

Intermittent openings in the walls led from the path into individual family compounds. We entered our first compound onto a scene that repeated itself many times over the next three days. The team leader spoke in Hausa to the women in the household to exchange greetings, explain our purpose and obtain permission for us to look at arms. The women smiled and tipped their heads toward me. I returned their greeting the same way.

Most women wore flimsy T-shirts with their wrappers of cotton print, colors dulled by hard wear and bright sun. In these private quarters, women didn't have to hide their hair with turbans. Their numerous braids formed intricate designs.

On two sides of the typical courtyard, window and door openings in the wall revealed individual rooms. It appeared much of life happened in the open-air common area, and our presence did not seem to impact its pace. Women pounded grain in a stone mortar, cooked or washed clothes and dishes. A large cast iron cauldron sat on a fire pit. Wet laundry was laid out on anything that would elevate it off the dirt. One of the women bent forward at a ninety-degree angle and swept the courtyard's dirt floor with a short-handled handmade broom. Teenage girls braided hair.

Older children took care of younger ones. I observed, as I had elsewhere, African children are seldom fussy. An older sibling or adult seems to anticipate and supply every need before it's expressed. In many African cultures, when children reach puberty, they go through a rite of passage and are then expected to assume adult responsibilities: a child one day and an adult the next. The young children played games in the dirt and shared without protest their toys handmade from wood, animal hide and feathers.

Socioeconomic class was evident. The best houses had two-foot-thick walls to keep the occupants cooler, and tapestry or pieces of carpet provided decor. Their mud-mound ovens were larger. The presence of more wives distinguished a select few compounds as belonging to the affluent. (Muslim men are permitted four wives, provided they can pay the bride price and afford to take care of those they marry.)

By midmorning the wall-enclosed paths trapped and concentrated the heat. We had started our day at seven, and I had forgotten to bring water. As the temperature climbed, I tried to ignore the open sewers' stench. I maneuvered to fend off the attacks of the fly population, but because the people around me did not react to flies crawling on their lips or even on the mucosa around their eyes, I tried to be subtle in my personal battle.

We followed the path dictated by the statistical grid. We checked arms. We documented. We moved on.

In the early afternoon, we came to the last compound for the day. It appeared to belong to a man at the pinnacle of Old City society. Our team leader once again interpreted for me from Hausa. The family wanted us to wait for the husband to arrive and ask his permission to check for scars. They brought out stools and placed them in the one niche of the courtyard where thatch provided a spiderweb of shade. I welcomed the relief for my feet and thankfully accepted a Fanta orange soda pop. Rather than satisfy my desire to interact and get to know a little more about this family, I followed the team's example and remained silent and unobtrusive.

The children in this household played with mass-produced plastic toys. One little girl had a bright green plastic doll like the one Meninge had bought for Ginger. A couple of girls, perhaps about eight years of age, tended to the many younger children.

Seeing the woman identified as the first wife (I had thought she was the grandmother), my impression was of a woman deemed too old, too infirm or too respected—perhaps all the above—to do any work. One of the children brought her a drink, stayed close and attended to any request.

The second and third wives, wearing their cotton wrappers, prepared food. One pounded grain in a stone mortar with a four-foot-long wooden pestle that made a weighty thud with each strike. The other stood at a large cauldron simmering with enough groundnut soup for thirty people and stirred with a wooden paddle almost as tall as she, releasing its enticing aroma. The muscled arms of both women reflected a life of hard physical labor.

Three feet from me in the favored alcove, a rich-looking carpet covered the dirt floor in front of the occupant of a deeply carved wooden chair upholstered with brocade. Clouds of organdy—lavender and yellow gossamer—enveloped the thirteen-year-old body of the fourth wife. She wore gold bangles and gold rings with brilliant stones. Gold earrings and necklaces shone against perfect ebony skin. This princess-like child had but to look in the direction of a cold bottle of Fanta or the large ostrich feather fan for others to immediately attend her. She did not talk or engage with anyone. As far as I could tell, she did not make eye contact with us or with anyone else. Her eyes seemed to look off in the distance, at nothing in particular. Her fixed half smile never changed.

We waited about twenty minutes before the husband walked through the doorway. Embroidery covered his kufi and the borders of his expansive robe. He was rotund and friendly, even jovial. Addressing me in British English, he apologized for delaying us and said that of course we could check his family. Then this sixtyish-looking man squared his shoulders and beamed with apparent pride as he strode over to his child bride. We completed our look at the arms in his household and ended our first day.

As we made our way along the maze of paths back to the front gate at around two o'clock, I patted the camera tucked deep in the pocket of my dress. I longed for a pictorial record I knew I would never have. A camera changes relationships. Photos weren't worth the cost.

# 29

# HOLD THE CELEBRATION

*Everyone in our* program had been preparing for the big announcement—that all of Nigeria was smallpox-free. But on March 20, down in Kaduna, a fourteen-year-old Yoruba girl was admitted to the infectious disease hospital—and the diagnosis was confirmed.

No question about it. Smallpox.

Reinforcements from other areas descended on her home village in Kwara State, and SMP personnel, including EIS officers, were rushed there from Atlanta. Carl and his teams redoubled their surveillance activities in Kano State, and the other operations officers and medical epidemiologists blitzed through their areas as well, especially all across the northern tier of states.

They contained the outbreak in short order. An amazing team.

# 30

# THE VOID

*New Year's Day* had come and gone, and a new decade had arrived. This time I hadn't thought about New Year's resolutions, or a neglected area in my life. When we decided to move to Africa, Carl and I had known we would miss our home church. But we were determined to keep up regular Bible study and Christian worship in our home if we didn't find a church family in Kano. Yes. Without fail.

When our first Sunday morning in Africa came, we'd been preparing to have our service when a friend stopped by and invited us to join them for a fun morning at the Kano Club—or something. Well, okay, we would have our service in the evening. At the end of a day of fun and too much sun, we were worn out and the kids were sleepy. We hurriedly read a few Bible verses, sang a couple of songs, prayed a prayer and rushed through our communion.

The next Sunday came. It went the same way. Since the other Americans planned a schedule full of diversions on Sundays, we always had invitations. For a few months, we did these quick worship services on Sunday nights. But we were usually too tired or distracted to focus. It became an afterthought. Then, one

Sunday night, we just forgot. And that was it—the end of it. The beginning of forgetting.

With neglecting our Sunday worship, we also neglected Bible study and prayer. I can't say whether Carl continued private prayer, but I left that out too. I hadn't made a decision to leave God out of my life. I just gradually allowed distractions to crowd him out.

In a few years, we would both return to our spiritual roots. Thanks to God's grace and mercy, our Christian life would be stronger than ever. But in Africa I stopped connecting with God just when I would need him most.

# 31

## A FATEFUL DECISION

*"I can't believe* it. It's like a Hollywood set," I remember saying. I was looking over Carl's shoulder at the brochure that March afternoon in 1970.

"Yeah, B-B, but that's beside the point." Carl always arched one eyebrow to emphasize a point (but also when skeptical or annoyed). "Main thing is, I'm needed there immediately."

Equatorial Guinea, one of West Africa's three Guineas, had recently gained its independence from Spain and wanted the smallpox/measles program there. CDC's Atlanta office added EG to the other nineteen countries in the program, and needed an operations officer who could speak Spanish. It would take valuable months to recruit and train a new person. They put out a call for an officer already on board in West Africa who could transfer there in a few weeks.

Before I knew anything about it, Carl had volunteered to go. (In the early years of our marriage, he made decisions like that for our lives, always driven by what he believed was the right thing to do. And in those days, rather consistent with my upbringing, I didn't push back.)

Nigeria had been a mesmerizing introduction to Africa. The hypnotic and the disturbing intermingled. We savored the experience and expected to stay in Kano a full two years. But now, after just eight months, we'd have to move on.

The next six weeks passed in a hurry. Carl finalized his work. He checked on the readiness of isolation facilities in the towns and isolation huts in the bush. He and the teams worked longer hours. They showed the smallpox identification photo from village to village, even house to house. Had anyone seen a person with these symptoms? Carl was gratified to find no new smallpox cases. But he doubled down on review of search-and-containment procedures with his teams. Continued vigilance was paramount. Through the program's continued surveillance, it would later be established that there were no new cases anywhere in Nigeria after May 1970, our last month there.

A few years had passed since we'd used our Spanish, so we sped through a review. The State Department sent us the seven-tape foreign service language course, and the US Information Service loaned us a big Wollensak reel-to-reel tape player.

I braved the tangle of traffic, scurried over to Sarki Trader and acquired a few more masks, drums and stools. I visited the palace one last time. And I finally witnessed a large camel caravan come in off the Sahara, a sight rapidly fading into history. My camera was at home.

I got our boxes ready. Adamu wanted to help, and did, but there was little to pack. We had the few things we'd been allowed to bring by air, plus African art now, including five brass mortar and pestle sets. Our full household shipment from home still floated somewhere on the Atlantic, or was in some West African port or other. Our red Volkswagen Beetle had arrived two weeks before, and we sold it, as we would have no use for a car in Santa Isabel (now Malabo), a town barely over one mile square.

Caesar, a big Siamese cat, had deigned to accept our hospitality and would have to be transported. Another expat family sold us a wire cage at a good price—probably the same family who had pushed us to adopt the feline in the first place.

We grabbed spare minutes to delve into the brochure and briefing about our new home: a change from the dry, dusty, dull brown, wide-open Sahel, to a dense tropical jungle with brilliant emerald greens sparkling against deeper green rain forest and the white froth of waterfalls. From heat-crackling dry air to skin-enhancing moisture. I pinched myself as I studied the photos and reread the glowing narrative.

The brochure showed the island of Fernando Po (now Bioko), tucked up tight into the sharp curve of the West African coast—the armpit, someone said. A quaint little capital, Santa Isabel was enchantment itself with its Spanish architecture and red tile roofs. Black sand beaches and a volcano supplied a dramatic setting for the tiny town. Bordered by the presidential palace and the twin towers of a neo-Gothic cathedral, the plaza sat above the perfect semicircle of a harbor, its arms embracing the deep sapphire-blue water. Colorful birds called this their home. The world's finest cacao grew from the rich black volcanic topsoil on the lush plantations, the brochure said, and the local fishing industry provided abundant fresh fish. The area was noted for its shrimp and their larger cousins, the prawns. A stereotypical tropical island paradise.

The rest of Equatorial Guinea was made up of scattered tiny islands and islets, and a speck of mainland squeezed between Gabon and Cameroon. And it was home to 260,000 warm and friendly people. It sounded idyllic. I had loved Africa so far, and it was about to get even more fascinating.

Besides all that, the US had a little embassy there, so someone could proctor my board exams. With my master's and the clinical fellowship year behind me, when I passed the national boards, I'd have my certificate of clinical competence, my "C's."

Despite having to say good-bye to our new friends in Kano, my sense of adventure and Carl's tug to serve where no one else would, continued to grow. Yes, we knew malaria, yellow fever and a whole range of other tropical hazards lurked within the romantic tropical setting, but vaccinations and knowledge had fortified us against those.

The movers came and picked up our boxes. With luck, they would arrive in Santa Isabel before we did. We found other employers for Adamu, Audu and Shetima, and, of course, Musa. Adamu wanted to stay with the USAID house, as the servant quarters there were nicer for his family than most alternatives. I think he counted on a new tenant's responding to his infectious smile just as we had. Living out of suitcases generated few messes in the house, but we kept all the men on the payroll until their new jobs began. They had been such a part of our lives. It wouldn't be easy to say good-bye.

Rounds of dinners in the homes of our Indian and American friends kept us busy. We would leave in eight more days.

---

"Hey, Carl? You here?" Tom Antorietto, a good friend by now, called through the screen door. "I've got an urgent message for you from the embassy."

I shot a puzzled look at my husband. Our program communications always came from the SMP regional office in Lagos, or maybe from USAID, not directly from the State Department. Carl was to go to Tom's office, where he could have a secure communication with the American embassy in Lagos. He grabbed a notepad and pen and headed out the door with Tom.

Hmm—a bit ominous. Carl hadn't mentioned any concerns at the new post, and Equatorial Guinea hadn't even been mentioned when we were in Atlanta. Oh, yes. Except for that puzzling comment made by our friend, that he would never consider an assignment to EG. He obviously had not changed his mind.

I waited. You do a lot of waiting when there are no phones and the nearest teletype or two-way radio communication device is several miles away. I read a few stories to the kids and put them to bed. Then I picked up my book and stared at a page. Carl returned an hour after he left.

I jumped up when I heard the crunch of gravel and met him at the door. "What's this about? Problem?"

Carl told me that State said he needed to fly down to Lagos and spend a couple of days at the embassy reading the cable traffic coming from the embassy in Equatorial Guinea. "They want to be sure I'm making an informed—"

"A fine time!" I slammed the book shut, angry at some absent bureaucrat. If there was a problem, why wait till now to bring it up? Before our things shipped would have been nice!

I said it was a little on the scary side. Carl was sure they were just being cautious. He stuffed a few items into an overnight bag and early the next day headed for the airport.

He returned from Lagos two days later, rushed, preoccupied, and a bit more mysterious than usual. He just said there wasn't time to give me a lot of detail about his meetings. Carl held a high-level clearance. He'd met with I-don't-know-who, and maybe he'd been in talks he could never reveal.

What he did tell me was he'd been shown a stream of cable traffic coming out of the US embassy in Santa Isabel. That sublime tropical island paradise was in the iron grip of a dictator named Francisco Macias Nguema. Under pressure from the United Nations, Spain had rushed through the process to grant independence. With too few noticing or caring, a sly, corrupt candidate people thought couldn't possibly win the country's first presidential election did. By now his reign of terror was well underway, and the country was cut off from journalistic reporting.

Cable after cable detailed the dictator's capricious torture and arbitrary killings.

In one bizarre episode at the stadium, the diplomatic corps witnessed Macias's executions of supposed subversives, including one horribly bungled hanging, to the accompaniment of "Those Were the Days," the Mary Hopkins hit song. (He would later repeat this grotesque display on Christmas Eve, 1975, when he executed 150 supposed coup plotters, the same song blaring over the loudspeakers, and his executioners dressed in Santa Claus costumes.)

In the recent past, gangs of armed youth had roamed the streets, beating the unfortunates who happened to be in their path.

But nine embassies and diplomatic missions jockeyed for influence and elbow room in the strategically located one-square-mile capital city. Russia and its allies were popular with the dictator and gaining ground every day, while America had no prestige there. Fielding the smallpox-measles program would give the US a foot in the door.

The latest cables indicated that curfews and other measures had been effective, and "calm had been largely restored."

Our family would be four of the six Americans resident in Equatorial Guinea. The State Department wanted to be sure Carl was fully briefed. Was he still willing to go there? He had closed out his work in Kano. What else could he do? His solution to the dilemma was to go on alone, feel the pulse of the country, and talk with the diplomats and United Nations people posted there. Then he would decide what we would do.

He packed for a known destination but an unknown length of stay. He drummed his fingers on any nearby surface as he hurriedly talked himself through each decision of what to take or not take.

Carl arrived in Equatorial Guinea on April 30, 1970. He had no way to communicate directly with me but would send a cable once he made the decision.

I waited with the kids and our suitcases.

A week later, Tom was at our door again. The conversations "on the ground" had convinced Carl that The Terror, as it was known, would not be directed at foreign diplomats or foreign aid workers. The American chargé d'affaires in Santa Isabel and the ambassador who was accredited there assured Carl we would be safe. So he gave the green light for us to join him.

Relieved, I stuck a box of crayons, the green plastic doll and the last few changes of clothes into the luggage. Now that I actually might need the information, I tucked my State Department protocol guide into my tote bag. The next day, May 8, 1970, Charles and Ginger and I boarded the Nigerian Airways VC-10 and headed for the tropical island pictured in the brochure.

# PART II

# IF YOU SCREAM
# AND NOBODY HEARS . . .

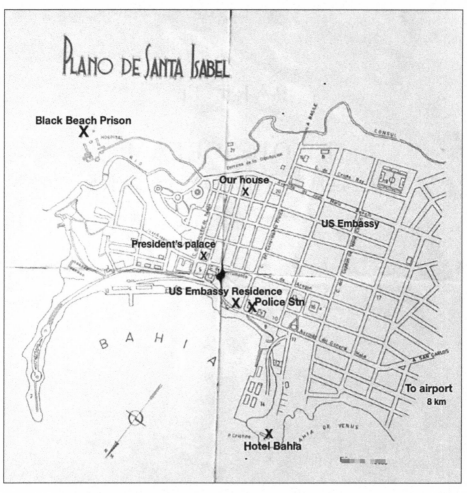

Street map of Santa Isabel, approximately one square mile

# 1

# MR. AMBASSADOR

*As the crow* flies, Santa Isabel, Equatorial Guinea, sits fewer than six hundred miles from Kano, Nigeria, but it was like a world away. The trip from Anglophone Africa through Francophone Africa to the only Spanish-speaking country in sub-Saharan Africa required three flights and three travel days. Happily, Charles, now a big five-year-old, and even Ginger, just turned two, were good travelers. Smallpox colleagues hosted us and our cat Caesar in Lagos the first night, sending us off the next day for our flight to Douala, Cameroon.

The US vice consul greeted us in Douala, his high-pitched voice piercing through the airport hubbub. He helped us through customs and said he'd drive us to the hotel where the consulate had reserved our room for the night.

As he maneuvered his car through the chaos of bicycles, cars, trucks and crowds of pedestrians, I expected him to say something like, "I can't believe you're going to a place like Equatorial Guinea," or at least, "Good luck." Maybe he was too busy avoiding pedestrians and crashes and making good use of the horn, but he didn't say a word about trouble there. I had to ask. He seemed nonchalant. Yes, President Macias was a bad guy, but his actions weren't directed at outsiders, and I didn't need to worry. Besides—over the past month calm had been largely restored on the island. There was that phrase again. Calm restored.

Well, okay, maybe Carl had overreacted and misinterpreted, just a bit, when he read the cables in Lagos. Being so serious-minded, he could worry about his family too much at times. Yeah. That was it. After all, this vice consul probably read daily cable traffic too. I could relax. And our children were so young that any difficulties we might have surely wouldn't affect them.

At the hotel, our escort said he would take us back to the airport the next morning. After he checked us in and was heading for the door, he said over his shoulder that, by the way, Ambassador Hoffacker would be flying over to the island with us tomorrow. It was time for his quarterly visit.

I had never met an ambassador and tomorrow I had to travel with one! Now where did I put that protocol guide? I only skimmed the confusing calling card etiquette that went something like, "When calling on a person of higher rank, e.g. an ambassador's wife, place the card on the silver tray provided. If calling in person, turn down the card's upper right corner." Then came many details about which corner to turn down to convey which message, and when to place what initials on the card.

But calling card protocol wasn't going to help me tomorrow. I had to get this Foreign Service stuff straight—learn some titles at least. I'd have questions in the morning.

The hotel's front desk had paper. I had crayons. These would occupy part of our evening. We had some dinner and settled in. Caesar meowed furiously. We let him out of his cage and gave him the run of the room. I read a couple of books to the kids, settled them into bed and then tried to sleep. What was that about the ambassador's "visiting" the embassy? I didn't understand.

## May 10, 1970

I got some answers on the way to the airport. Since Santa Isabel was such a small post, Ambassador Lew Hoffacker was accredited to both Cameroon *and* Equatorial Guinea. His resident embassy was in Yaoundé, Cameroon, and he visited the embassy in Santa Isabel once a quarter, staying four or five days each time. Chargé d'Affaires Al Williams was the person in charge in Santa Isabel except during the ambassador's visits.

I felt a little nervous and must have wiped the perspiration from the back of my neck as we approached the airport. Even an ambassador's full title is intimidating: Ambassador Extraordinary and Plenipotentiary.

When we arrived at the airport, Ambassador Hoffacker was deep in conversation with the US Consul. He looked pretty serious. Under his wire-rimmed glasses and every-hair-in-place coif, his expression was one I couldn't read. Maybe it was the blank diplomatic mask I'd heard people talk about.

I took a deep breath. I could do this.

I needn't have worried. When the ambassador looked up and spotted us, he came over and introduced himself. Through his professional reserve, I sensed a gentleness. He asked how I was and how our trip had been so far and then excused himself to finish his business.

We waited for our way-behind-schedule flight. A man nearby said, "Their usual, I'd bet. Engine trouble."

When the ambassador picked up his carry-ons and joined us again, I remember my surprise at the large basket he carried. I had to know. "Excuse me, Mr. Ambassador, but I'm puzzled. Why are you taking all those green vegetables to Santa Isabel? In the pictures the island looks so lush."

He explained that the island was too lush. Too wet to grow

vegetables. He said that on each trip he carried as much as possible for the embassy—along with French cheeses from Cameroon.

We finally boarded our little Convair 440, one of two planes leased from Iberia Airlines to Equatorial Guinea for their fledging airline. The twenty-two-minute flight took us past volcanic Mt. Cameroon and out over twenty miles of the Atlantic Ocean toward our new home.

We and the four or five other passengers had barely settled in before the plane started its descent. Princesa, the only flight attendant for the airline's two planes, dashed up and down the aisle and thrust cups of some liquid, I don't remember what, into our hands. I hurried to finish with the cup, grabbed my compact and did a quick check in the mirror.

So excited now. Through the scratched window I searched the horizon.

Dense layers of rain forest and coastal coconut palms hid much of the island as we approached. Then we banked, and I saw on the left side of the plane a perfect semicircle of a bay and charming little town. Just like the brochure. Santa Isabel sat behind its crater harbor, looking like a single jewel set into a tiara.

We touched down on a runway bordered by banana trees on the inland side. Beyond them rose a high wall of rain forest, dense and the darkest green I'd ever seen.

As our plane taxied to a stop, I spotted a black embassy car, slowly covering the few dozen yards from the terminal to our plane. An American flag lightly rippled on the diplomatic flagstaff on the chauffeur-driven Chevy Nova. As the uniformed embassy driver emerged from the front, a man in his early thirties, close to my age, with black curly hair, bounced out onto the tarmac. And then I could see Carl through the window! But he looked so different. His beard was gone! He followed the stairs as they were wheeled up to the plane.

I felt sure we were supposed to wait until Ambassador Extraordinary and Plenipotentiary went down the steps before we started to deplane. But Ambassador Hoffacker insisted the kids and I deplane first. He extended his hand to carry my bags.

"Oh no, Mr. Ambassador! Please. I've got them."

"No. I insist." It was a flat statement of fact.

I gathered the loose items and led Charles and Ginger down the steps into a hot, saturating mist and into Carl's hugs, which never felt so good. I stroked the smooth chin. Carl's mom would be thrilled, but I was disappointed. I'd become fond of that beard.

Chargé d'Affaires Al Williams welcomed Ambassador Hoffacker while our family continued with big hugs and chatter all around. (Oh—but now that the ambassador's foot had touched the ground, and until he departed, Al would be the deputy chief of mission, not chargé. Right, Bee?) Now Al turned to us with a convivial smile and expansive gestures.

"Welcome to Santa Isabel, Bee! We're delighted you're here!" He said his wife, Carman, was eager to meet me. Until my arrival she'd been the only American woman in the country. I would meet her tonight at the embassy's reception for the ambassador.

Too soon, the welcome and our noisy reunion were quashed by a crisis with our very large cat. Several soldiers in dark green fatigues, eyes wide and legs braced, surrounded his wire cage. His Highness, Caesar, a cross between a short-hair Siamese and a long-hair Siamese, flaunted his regalness. The soldiers trained their dirty rifles on him, no doubt frightening our children and convincing them their pet was about to be killed.

Caesar, with arched back, tail fluffed, and adrenaline surging, puffed himself up into his most fearsome size, eyes ablaze, and his "khhhhhh" audible. I heard one of the soldiers mention a *"leon."* Were these the "calm restored" soldiers? Carl had Charles and Ginger by the hand. He nudged my elbow with his, signaling me to follow suit as he stepped back a couple of steps to let the professionals handle the situation.

Al Williams, obviously a skilled diplomat where cats were concerned, cheerily calmed the frightened men. My Spanish couldn't keep up with all the conversation, but anyone could have interpreted Al's chuckles as he drew the soldiers under his spell. He convinced them Caesar was not a lion and would not escape and attack. After more palaver and congenial laughs all around, we were allowed to proceed.

As the driver held the car door for the ambassador, I said, "It was a privilege to meet you, Mr. Ambassador," and I thanked him for his help. He really was an ordinary man after all.

The diplomats drove away as our family followed the soldiers toward the shed that served as a terminal. Carl whispered in my ear, "We'll be okay."

We stepped into the musty interior. Even in the dim light, I could see that no one smiled, neither soldiers nor passengers. We were on official passports, which made the immigration and customs process a little easier. Two men from our flight—one at a time—were rudely herded into a room off to the side.

Soldiers followed them into the room. Slammed the door shut.

# 2

# CALVO SOTELO

*When we finally* emerged from the terminal, the children and I joined Carl in the smallpox program's Dodge Power Wagon for the drive toward our next home.

Heading away from the airport for the eight-kilometer drive into town, ten-thousand-foot Pico Santa Isabel rose somewhere to our right, but the rain forest, so close to the road, and the cottony mist blocked our view. The brochure did not exaggerate the beauty of the island of Fernando Po.

Santa Isabel's outskirts, although "outskirts" seemed a misnomer relative to a town of little more than one square mile, revealed a cluster of shacks, then a collection of low concrete houses, and then, in the center of town, Spanish architecture graced by fan palms. Broken roof tiles marred the scene here and there, and iron grillwork encased a few empty balconies and windows.

We didn't have to fight the West Africa city traffic I'd gotten used to. So few vehicles or pedestrians here. So little noise. The streets were empty except for soldiers standing around. Where were all the people?

Carl said he would show us the harbor in a day or two, but for now we would go straight to the house, which he was sure I would like. And we needed to get ready to attend a reception and dinner for the ambassador.

From the edge of the "city limits," we had driven not more than a dozen city blocks before we parked in front of our corner house at 18 Calle de Calvo Sotelo. (I still have the sign the government tore down when they were ridding the country of all Spanish names.) The house had a tropical bungalow look. More modern than the Spanish colonial houses, its dark brown eaves, shutters and doors accented the white walls. We were about four blocks from that picturesque circular bay I'd seen from the air. Beyond our house, Calvo Sotelo extended only to the end of our long block. There, the edge of town met the edge of the rain forest, or at least the apron of the edge of the rain forest.

From the sidewalk in front of our house, a wrought-iron gate opened into the front yard and the short walkway to the pint-sized porch. Trees, shrubs and a hedge of green and deep red leaves gave privacy to the property. Dank, heavy air and pervasive moisture enveloped us.

Carl told me he had engaged a steward from among the many Nigerians here, and when the heavy front door opened, Samuel emerged. His gentle smile and melodious Igbo-accented English were as warm as the air.

"Oh, madame, welcome, welcome. And you sweet children. Come in and see your new home."

I liked Samuel immediately. His pleasant, quiet manner drew me in. Samuel had been highly recommended, and Carl trusted him. Over time, that trust would prove to be more than well placed.

The front door opened into a wide hallway leading straight back to the three bedrooms and bath. The entry's right wall of large gray stones curved around toward the living room, while at the same time forming one wall of the dining room.

"Carl! My goodness! This furniture!"

The Mediterranean style dining set and living room furniture with gold damask upholstery took me by surprise. Carl explained.

When furniture for the two houses arrived, Al and Carman didn't like this rather formal furniture. They wanted the casual rattan instead, so we had the furniture meant for the embassy. I laughed. Well, I guessed I could live with it.

One accessory in the living room was a surprise. A telephone. We really had a telephone. But it turned out we could call only other numbers here in this little town.

A long kitchen with ample cabinet space had easy access to both the living room and dining room. The back door opened from the kitchen onto a large covered concrete slab porch. I welcomed this as a protected area for Charles and Ginger to get some outdoor play during the frequent rains I'd read about. Beyond the porch, dozens of tropical plants—what other kind would there be?—stretched in straight rows across the back area. It looked like the former resident may have grown them to sell. The ground, moist to near saturation, supported a generous coat of moss and fungi. Fruit hung heavy on the banana tree and a couple of papaya trees.

I could not have been more pleased with the house and its grounds. And I had an early sense Samuel would be a perfect fit for our family. Carl had done well in getting it all set up for our arrival.

# 3

# STANDOFF

*While we were* dressing for the reception that evening, Carl told me about his first official act for the smallpox program here. His initial order of business, once he made the decision to stay, had been to meet with the minister of health, the man who would be his principal contact with the local government.

As chargé, Al Williams briefed Carl before this first meeting, but the minister's opening gambit was still a surprise. My fearless husband described the scene to me.

The minister locked eyes with him, pointedly placed his revolver on the desk between them, and held the eye contact to give time for that move to sink in. He then announced there would be no petrol for the smallpox/measles program vehicles.

If he were to enforce that, the program would never get off the ground.

Would Carl be stopped in his tracks like most other advisors this government requested? The United Nations expert on tropical agriculture had been invited into the country to assist, and then forbidden to visit a farm or even to talk to his local agriculture counterpart. After months of frustrated efforts, he gave up, resigned and left the country.

But Carl was his usual unflappable self. In his most indifferent manner, he told the minister the lack of petrol made no difference to him. He would just go to his house and spend his days napping and smoking cigars. The minister abruptly ended the meeting, but Carl left, confident in the effectiveness of his tactic. The next morning, he had all the petrol he needed, and he geared up immediately to begin operations.

The incident wasn't something to take lightly, but Carl got a big kick out of telling me this story. Just like with another encounter he'd tell me about some years later. A news crew got on his elevator in a near-empty hotel somewhere in—Central America, I think. For some reason unknown to me, he was once again in a country most Americans had evacuated. "What are *you* doing here?" the startled crew asked. He didn't answer.

# 4

# SO THIS IS THE FOREIGN SERVICE

*I had survived* traveling with the ambassador, but this evening's initiation into the world of diplomats and their soirées was another matter. I asked Carl what I should wear to a party for an ambassador.

"Well, from what I've seen so far, it'll be really casual. I wouldn't worry, B-B." He shot me a mischievous smile. "You'll look great no matter what you wear." I'd had a couple of new dresses made while we were in Kano. I would wear one of those.

We arrived as the cocktail hour got underway. And Carl was right. Dress couldn't have been more relaxed—festive, but casual and cool as suited the tropics. (And I would never need those calling cards.)

Carl seemed proud to introduce me around. Many in the group had heard about my arrival.

Our ambassador, the guest of honor, passed the evening deep in conversation with one cluster of guests after another. I could never read him. *There's a gentleness about him, but he has an expression that gives nothing away.*

Ambassador Hoffacker was a World War II combat veteran who'd been seriously wounded in Okinawa. I didn't know it then, but he'd been the US consul in Elizabethville, the Congo, in the midst of the first of the US–Soviet proxy wars in Africa. One night, when arriving with US Senator Thomas Dodd at a dinner he was hosting for the senator, he snatched two of three dinner guests—a United Nations representative and a Belgian banker— from the clutches of armed kidnappers and rushed them into the limo where Mrs. Dodd and his own wife, Connie, were sitting. After spiriting everyone back to the consulate, where they hoped for safety from the battle outside, he was on the telephone all night. By morning he had negotiated the release of the third kidnap victim, another UN representative, who was returned bloodied but alive. Many credited Ambassador Hoffacker with saving Senator Dodd's life. A tough sort despite the gentle exterior.

Next in the US diplomatic hierarchy was Al Williams—he who had negotiated the resolution of the cat crisis earlier in the day. He was a foreign service officer (FSO) of the tall, dark and suave variety and possessed one of those voices that sounds like its owner is smiling. He appeared to thoroughly enjoy people and was a good listener. Al glided among the other diplomats with casual grace and was never far from his next genial chuckle.

Carman Williams, Al's adept foreign service wife, vivacious and attractive, laughed an easy, delightful laugh that carried over the hum and buzz of a room full of conversations. It seemed to me she was always laughing, but not inappropriately. Her delighted-with-life smile crinkled the corners of her eyes, and her long blondish ponytail tossed about with the liveliness of her animated conversation. I decided Al and Carman could lift anybody's mood. Besides Carman's duties as first lady of the embassy, she served as the administrative officer for this, the smallest US embassy in the world.

Al and Carman were fluent in Spanish and French (Al also spoke Russian), and they had been transferred from Dakar,

Senegal, to open the embassy here. Their two children, ages ten and fourteen, I think, had remained in Dakar at their missionary school, now as boarding students. The other FSO at our embassy, Third Secretary J. Grant Burke, was a bachelor. He must have been lost in the crowd that night. I don't remember noticing him. I had now met all the official Americans, the entire permanent American population in Equatorial Guinea—three, not counting the visiting ambassador. Our family would make seven.

Diplomats from several countries, a few Equatorial Guinean officials and representatives from the Organization of African Unity (OAU) turned out to honor Ambassador Hoffacker. I met the French and Nigerian ambassadors and their wives, the ambassador from Cameroon, a counselor from the embassy of Ghana and his wife and Britain's honorary vice-consul. Heady company for a small-town gal like me. A handful of United Nations technical advisors from various Latin American countries rounded out the group. Knowing smiles and laughter seemed to erupt when anyone mentioned the Spanish ambassador. He was on home leave—and on his honeymoon.

The group greeted me enthusiastically. Any enlarging of the tiny social circle lifted the spirits. The wives in particular seemed thankful to have another woman around. I was awe-struck by everyone and everything. So this was the foreign service. I would waltz through the coming weeks on a giddy high, impressed that I was in such exalted company.

Over time I would realize the forced sparkle glossing over tension in a group of people living life on vigil.

# 5

## BUT IT LOOKS LIKE PARADISE

*It was May* 11, 1970, my first morning in Santa Isabel. Carl took me to see his office. We could have walked the five blocks, a straight shot from our house, but we were pressed for time.

Carl told me we would stay just a few minutes at the chancery. Then we would have to move on. What? The chancery? I thought this was the embassy. He had said his office was in the embassy.

"Same thing," Carl said. He explained that either word may refer to the offices, and the words "embassy" or "the residence" can refer to the official residence. He said that even ambassadors aren't consistent, so no need to stress over it.

Our chancery/embassy sat on a corner in a mixed neighborhood of homes and businesses. The red tile roof and open block work accented the two-story white Spanish colonial. The Great Seal of the United States and an American flag adorned the curving upstairs balcony.

In contrast, from the sidewalk Carl pointed up the street a half block. "The Russians stay inside their big concrete bunker of an embassy. If one of them goes to the store, it's never alone. They always go in pairs."

At our own friendly-looking chancery, a heavy front door led into a modest and spare reception area with its plain white walls.

A telephone and a lamp looked lonely on the unmanned desk. A few chairs for visitors, the American flag and the official portrait of President Nixon completed the decor. The hum of window air conditioners accompanied our tour.

Three small offices opened off the reception area. Inside Carman's office, a massive steel door led into a vault. The Williams's sweet poodle, Sarah, sat atop a diplomatic pouch.

On the second floor, a studio apartment awaited any temporary personnel, and an open area near the top of the stairs held Carl's desk and files. Double doors opened onto the balcony with access to the flag.

We didn't linger long at the chancery before heading to the *ayuntamiento* (city hall). Along with Ambassador Hoffacker, Al Williams and J. Grant Burke, we would be given an official tour. The mayor met us at the main entrance. As our guide, he talked at length and with pride about the functions of each city office as we proceeded through the muggy interior, a dank environment one could expect a block from the sea. We climbed the stairs to the second floor.

About twenty minutes into the tour, as the mayor explained yet another activity of the city, a second government official appeared at the door and motioned for him to step outside the room, which he did. He then reappeared in the doorway for a moment, excused himself, and left for several minutes. When he returned to our little group, he apologized for the interruption of our tour.

"I'm sorry to have to leave you. The president has just fired me." He was immediately led away.

After we were escorted from the building, we left the ayuntamiento and went to the residence for what the ambassador called a postmortem on the day's event. Carl and I listened to the diplomats discuss this as well as other bizarre occurrences.

They talked about the implications, political and otherwise, and about Americans' security here. I gathered they were making assumptions based on shards and shreds of intelligence gleaned by paying close attention. I remember they said we could feel safe. Knowing Carl, I'm sure he was checking my reaction. I wasn't frightened. I just couldn't believe what I had seen and heard, and felt something akin to exhilaration that I was allowed to listen in on this conversation.

And I had this strange feeling—as though I had landed in a fictional place. It was more stage worthy than any scene I had imagined.

Then the conversation turned dark. The mayor's fate? He would likely disappear into Black Beach Prison and be tortured, maybe killed. He had incurred the president's displeasure—for some reason. Or no reason.

Tomorrow I would search through Carl's material on the history of Equatorial Guinea. I had to understand the past of this place.

—➤

Foreign policy leader Ambassador Raymond Garthoff would later have something to say about the embassy. From experience at RAND Corporation, the CIA, the Department of State, and in leading inspections of US embassies in Africa, he authored *A Journey through the Cold War: A Memoir of Containment and Coexistence*. He writes that most foreign missions departed Equatorial Guinea because of the pressures of the dictatorship, but that America "had decided to leave the two-man listening post."

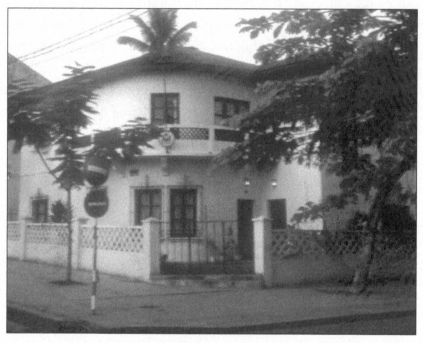

The US embassy chancery building, Santa Isabel,
Equatorial Guinea, 1970

# 6

# A LITTLE HISTORY

*Would I find* anything to shed light on the mayor's abrupt firing? I had only Carl's State Department and CIA fact sheets, his reports to CDC, and what the diplomats told us. Not much to go on.

Our friends back home asked, "Where exactly do you live?" and it's no wonder they were confused. There were two other Guineas in West Africa—Portuguese Guinea (later Guinea-Bissau) and Guinea (former French Guinea), neighbors to each other on the continent's great western bulge. Equatorial Guinea (former Spanish Guinea) sat under that shoulder in the curve where the continental coast turns south again.

The country had been unknown, ignored and isolated. Macias had closed down the press, expelled all journalists, prohibited importing of magazines and newspapers, seized control of radio and TV and censored all mail. Spain prohibited any mention of its former colony in the press—declared it a violation of the State Secrets Act. The cryptic notes I would make about our day-to-day experiences, I'd keep well hidden in case the Guardia searched our house.

Colonial powers had cobbled this country together from diminutive, disparate and distant parts. Fernando Po, our home island, sat at three degrees north of the equator; Rio Muni, a speck of the continent, was at two degrees north; and remote, six-square-mile Annobon at one degree south. This was going to be a commute unlike any Carl had ever had.

Fernando Po and adjacent coasts were so disease ridden they had long been known as one of the unhealthiest places on earth—a white man's graveyard. Yellow fever and malaria were the most deadly. An outbreak of yellow fever a century earlier killed 78 of the 280 whites on the island.

"You and those kids will come home in a pine box!" Carl's parents said. They'd been furious when he'd broken the news we were moving to Africa.

Corseted in her Victorian dress, nineteenth-century English explorer Mary Kingsley waded through West Africa's swamps, tromped through steamy rain forests and recorded her rigorous observations. At one point she fell through the leafy camouflage of a deep pit onto sharp pointed stakes intended to kill. All those petticoats saved her life. In a vivid remark about Fernando Po's epidemics, she said that to be posted there as Spanish governor general was "equivalent to execution, only more uncomfortable in the way it worked out."

Our dozen mandatory vaccinations would protect us against yellow fever and more. We would stave off deadly malaria by use of mosquito repellent and netting and the bitter chloroquine tablets. Not easy for our toddler and preschooler to swallow. Boiled water and bleach-soaked produce completed our defense against the pine box scenario.

Control of this Slave Coast area had bounced back and forth among African tribes. After Portuguese explorers first discovered and claimed Fernando Po in the fifteenth century, the power over the island had gone to Portugal and then to Spain, Britain and back to Spain. A lot of that colonial ping-pong seemed to have to do with who most wanted slaves when.

I found it ironic that after centuries of benefiting from the slave trade, Britain leased the island of Fernando Po from Spain for the purpose of suppressing that trade. Tightly packed cargoes of Africans who had been captured by stronger tribes and sold to the slavers were set free, many of them at our beautiful little harbor.

When Britain's lease ended in 1844, Spain used this island as a convict colony. They transferred political prisoners from Spain and "rebellious" subjects from the colonies of Cuba and the Philippines. Now, besides suffering the harsh colonial rule, the native islanders saw these "outsiders" transform their neighborhood. Decades later, Spaniards came to the island as settlers and ruled with Francoist Spain's heavy hand.

Further tangled colonial deals gave Spain control of the other pieces of this country, and they christened the whole "Spanish Guinea." All of the bits together would fit inside the US state of Maryland with a little wiggle room left over. The reported population—260,000—was a complex ethnic mixture. Fang, Bubi, Fernandino, and Nigerian Igbo, along with several much smaller tribes, sparred for space. The mayor we'd seen fired and led away was Bubi, and Macias, the dictator, was Fang.

Carl would spend most of his time among the Fang, who occupied the majority of Rio Muni and constituted more than two thirds of Equatorial Guinean citizens, even before they killed off so many Bubi on Fernando Po. I didn't know at the time that *Encyclopedia Britannica* said, "the Fang fought their way to the sea in the 19th and early 20th centuries by subjugating other groups in their path." And they "cultivated their reputation" as cannibals to intimidate other tribes.

Cannibals! I don't know whether the Fang were really cannibals, and I'm thankful I didn't hear that rumor until later. Some historians say this was a myth an early nineteenth-century explorer started and passed along to other explorers. Traders who wanted to scare competitors away from their lucrative turf perpetuated it.

The Fang did practice witchcraft, and one Fang cult, the Bwiti, practiced human sacrifice. Bwiti ceremonies took place in the forest. At night. And required a corpse. When the group had no corpse for the ceremony, human sacrifice was employed to supply one. Another point of blissful ignorance for me at the time. One authority says the practice of human sacrifice was vanishing among the Bwiti in the 1970s.

Various witchcraft societies practiced necrophagy, eating specific parts of an admired, deceased person to assimilate desired qualities. A few sources indicate necrophagy had disappeared by the time we arrived. Well, even if eating a dead body hadn't completely disappeared when we were there in the early '70s, I'm pretty sure we didn't have the qualities that would have landed us on the menu.

The Bubi, early inhabitants of the island, had migrated there from the mainland. In their first contact with European diseases, their numbers had evidently been decimated until only fifteen thousand remained, and far fewer when we arrived, I believe. They were so small in number and so isolated that frequent albinism and other genetic mutations occurred. One of the Santa Isabel bank tellers had six fingers on each hand. The telegraph operator had none—and typed with only nubs.

The three thousand Fernandinos on the island were mixed-race descendants from the liberated slaves, other freedmen from Sierra

Leone and transplants from Cuba. Fernandinos had been the social and economic elite in the distant past. One of them, Ricardo (not his real name), was Carl's respected and highly valued administrative assistant.

Bubis and Fernandinos aspired to succeed in business, civil service or the professions, and Spain had favored them over the Fangs in granting educational opportunities. Many had traveled outside the country for higher education.

Outnumbering all the local tribes combined were seventy thousand Nigerians, mostly Igbos from the southeastern region. When the Spanish established their plantations on the island, they tried to divert the Bubis from cultivating and trading their traditional crop—yams—to working lucrative but labor-intensive cacao. When the Bubis couldn't be enticed, the Spanish contracted with Nigeria for laborers who brought their families and settled on the plantations or in tight communities in Santa Isabel. That population swelled as the Nigerian Civil War strangled the Biafra homeland.

Most Equatorial Guineans were nominally Roman Catholic, many mixing that faith with their native practices. The Catholic Church operated the hospitals. Up until independence and in the early months afterward, Catholics, some Baptists and a few other Protestant groups supplied many education and health-care services.

Spain was a harsh master, and any efforts by the Africans it ruled to free themselves from colonial rule were punished by imprisonment and torture or exile. Even though in 1959 it granted all Spanish Guinea's citizens, including Africans, the same rights as Spanish citizens, that didn't guarantee much under Franco's dictatorship.

But independence fever had spread throughout sub-Saharan Africa. Except for Portugal, other colonial powers had seen the writing on the wall and accepted the inevitable. When the United Nations put pressure on Spain in late 1967, the Spanish initiated a hasty process toward independence and convened a conference to facilitate drafting a constitution. Ten months later they had a constitution and held an election one month before independence. Francisco Macias Nguema, one of the Fang candidates, won the presidency. On October 12, 1968, ill-prepared little Spanish Guinea became the independent Republic of Equatorial Guinea.

The Bubi Union's leaders had fought hard for Fernando Po to be its own country, separated from the dreaded Fang, but lost that battle. They were the most pro-Spanish and feared that when Spanish rule ended, the Fang would invade their island. They were right.

There would be no nation building. The nickname "Death's Waiting Room," applied to the area in the past because of disease, would soon be applied for a different reason. When we arrived in 1970, this fragile country was barely eighteen months old.

My dream of Africa had been one of living among the native peoples, not in an American bubble. The ambassador assured us the events here would not affect our safety, and the brochure talked about the warm and friendly people. I determined I would get acquainted with everyday Guineans.

# 7

## EERIE SILENCE

*May 12, 1970.* After breakfast we stepped into a mildew-tinged steamy day, the mist not heavy enough to fall in drops. Umbrella in hand, Charles, Ginger and I set out to explore Santa Isabel.

Nothing was far away in this town of barely over one square mile. We'd gone one block west and one block north when we found the first shop, a meager inventory on its shelves. Were they going out of business?

Seeing no other customers, I browsed through the few things they did have—festive beauty products and accessories from Spain and Portugal, more colorful than the English products in Nigeria. The elaborate Spanish hair combs and the dancer silhouetted in the red and black packaging of Maja perfumes reminded me of stories we read in high school Spanish class. Nothing had sounded more romantic than a senorita with the high comb and a mantilla. I bought shampoo and a new hairbrush. I'd be able to buy beauty products here, but not much else.

The next several shops were shuttered and appeared abandoned. Past those we stepped into a mercantile. Among their limited selection of fabrics, I found an open weave in a forest green for curtains to complement our dark wood shutters and window casings. I would return after I measured.

More vacant shop windows stared out of faded green, or dingy, whitewashed buildings. Graceful Spanish arches, colonnades and heavy wrought iron grillwork tried but failed to mask water-stained and moldy walls.

We came to a *farmacia*. Carman had said two of the four drugstores had closed and Macias now prohibited Western medicines as un-African. The proprietor looked bored. I didn't see much behind his counter, and he had run out of aspirin and Band-Aids, the only two things I planned to buy. As the locals might say, "It's all gone—finish."

Anticipating an opportunity to practice Spanish and get acquainted with my new community, I had trotted out my "Buenos dias. Como esta?" at each stop. Sadly for me, none of the merchants were the chatty sort. They were polite but subdued. They weren't busy with other customers. I knew most shop owners were Portuguese, but they'd served a Spanish clientele for decades and must have understood my simple greeting. And where were all the people?

I entered the grocer's, eager to see what I could or couldn't buy in Santa Isabel. Charles and Ginger could choose a treat to enjoy as we continued our stroll.

"*Buenos dias. Como esta usted?*"

A somber nod.

The door opened. Oh good—at least now there were a couple of other shoppers.

"*Buenos dias. Como estan ustedes?*"

I couldn't understand the mumbled response as they turned away.

We approached the tall wooden counter that stretched the length of the store. Behind it, floor-to-ceiling wooden shelves lined the wall. The wide spacing of the canned goods could not disguise the bareness. Fresh produce consisted of plantains and pineapple. What had Ambassador Hoffacker said—it's too wet to grow vegetables? I pointed to a couple of tins of green beans, and Charles and Ginger each chose a piece of candy.

We passed the post office. Nothing happening there.

Still hardly a car in sight on the streets. And the four or five Africans we passed on the sidewalk? Their gaze went to their feet or off into the distance. *I think that woman just crossed the street to avoid passing anywhere near me! What's going on? How silent and empty this place.*

And I suddenly realized something else—no music. It wasn't just the absence of voices and laughter, car horns and bicycle bells. I heard no rhythms of drums or chants. No mellow tones from flute or thumb piano coming from any of the businesses or shanties. Just silence.

When Mary Kingsley visited here a hundred years ago, she said the "sleepiness infected the [one] café and took all the go out of it." I didn't yet know it, but what I was beginning to sense now was nothing so benign as sleepiness.

After this two-block business district, the street ended at the coast road, so we turned east toward the plaza. I wanted to find a bench near the water. Maybe if other moms and their children were there, the children would break the ice. Charles and Ginger could start learning Spanish and get acquainted with games Spanish or African children play.

After two blocks, the street opened onto the Plaza de la Independencia. This square fronted the deep circular bay created by a sunken volcanic crater, its collapsed north rim forming the harbor mouth. Palm-fringed hundred-foot cliffs were its slender arms. With the once-a-month ship not at the dock, it was a curiously empty harbor. I had a perfect view of the blue jewel of a bay. The Spanish neo-Gothic cathedral with its twin towers sat on the plaza's west side. The presidential palace sat on the south side, opposite the harbor.

But the people. Where were the people? No comings and

goings at the cathedral. No one sitting or strolling by the water. Such a beautiful place. How could the plaza be empty?

I was relieved and delighted when, at last, two women and their two-year-old daughters arrived at the plaza. The moms and I visited, in Spanish. The children eyed each other for a while before any interaction. The women were from Spain. One said she also had a six-year-old and he was in school in Spain, living with grandparents. There were no children here Charles's age, she told me. In fact, almost no Spanish children lived in Santa Isabel now, and these two families were packing up to leave.

We sat and talked, and our children played together right in front of the palace of Macias Nguema. No people entered or left or lingered around the presidential enclave. The palace just sat there—leering.

I enjoyed the visit and the view in any direction except toward the palace, but it was time to get ready for a luncheon at the embassy residence. The children and I walked home. One block west and three blocks south.

At the end of Ambassador Hoffacker's five-day visit, the Williamses hosted a private luncheon for him with just the seven resident Americans.

I relayed my experience exploring the town and received answers to questions.

If local people crossed the street to avoid me, they had good reason. Four months ago, President Macias placed a ban on Equatorial Guineans having any contact with a foreigner. No one would risk the slightest appearance of interacting with us.

Yes, a lot of shops are empty and boarded up. A few months back, the youth militia demolished and looted most of them. They grabbed all the liquor and smashed counters and windows. The few shops that could reopen are pretty empty because there's almost no market now for their products. Most of the eight thousand Spaniards have been evacuated over the past several months.

The Portuguese shop owners aren't unfriendly; they're just depressed.

And Spanish mothers and children? Gone in the evacuation, home to Spain. Maybe a handful still here. The Spaniards were prime targets because they were the former colonial power, and the president hates the Spanish.

How much of this luncheon topic did Charles absorb? He was a smart five-year-old.

Ambassador Hoffacker said the Spaniards had good reason to evacuate, but the government here wouldn't bother us. They wouldn't attack foreign aid personnel or diplomats.

I didn't understand everything Al and the ambassador were talking about, but I got the impression that we should do a lot of listening in Santa Isabel. The next time we went out, I'd pay closer attention.

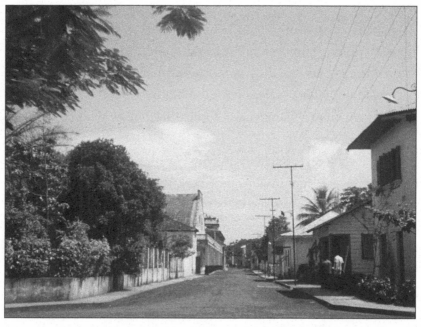

Eerily empty street viewed from in front of our house,
Santa Isabel, 1970

# 8

# AND THEN THERE WERE SIX

*It was late* and I really needed to go to bed—but I couldn't sleep after the day I'd had. The date was May 24, 1970, and I'd arrived in this tropical paradise exactly two weeks earlier. Carl was with his teams over on the mainland, so our embassy's Third Secretary, J. Grant Burke, phoned and offered to take the kids and me for a drive to see something outside of this one-square-mile town. He said we'd drive down the coast to the fishing village at San Carlos Bay. Absolutely. We'd love to go. The brochure about this country had promoted the thriving fishing industry, and the coastal waters "teeming with fish"—"renowned for shrimp and prawns," it said. If we stopped for lunch today, I knew what I would order!

The Atlantic was on our right. Cacao *fincas* (plantations) and tangled rain forest hugged the left shoulder. But rain forest also crept onto abandoned fincas. Passing a few scattered Bubi villages along the way, we covered two-thirds the length of the island in a leisurely hour. I watched for the boats. Halfway down the coast road, I concluded they must all be in port at San Carlos (now Luba) today, or maybe fishing on the other side of the island.

At *Bahia de San Carlos* (San Carlos Bay), I still saw no boats.

"Where's the thriving fishing industry?"

"Gone," Grant told me. People had been fleeing Equatorial

171

Guinea in droves, so President Macias ordered all the boats destroyed—either burned or sunk, depending on whose version you listened to—to prevent escape from the island. No more fishing industry.

No fishing boat, no little motor launch, no canoe. All gone. Just gone. We foreigners could fly out, but the locals were effectively incarcerated on the island.

At the beach in San Carlos, we went to a little thatch-covered outdoor café—the only café so far as I could tell. We had a wide choice of tables because the patio was deserted except for a couple of weathered and weary-looking expats. Spattered shade offered a bit of relief from the heat, but no breeze—just steamy air. The manager (Grant said he was the honorary German consul) took our order. The few foreigners left in the country like to come on Sundays for pink gin, but Charles and Ginger and I ordered *limonadas*. I was thinking any day with a lemonade by the sea is a good day.

But the day wasn't over yet.

We drove back up the coast, and Grant took us to our house. Taped on our front door was a note from Carman Williams, in large, urgent scrawl.

"Grant—come to Embassy immediately. Bee, we'll need you this p.m. too."

We hurried to the chancery. Al and Carman Williams were rushing about the office, elbow-deep in paper.

"Grant, you've been PNG'd!" (declared persona non grata). President Macias had given his ultimatum that morning, and Grant had twenty-four hours to leave the country. At least four of those hours were already gone. Al had called the president and asked him to explain his reason but got nowhere. Macias didn't need reasons.

Grant and Al huddled in the vault. I assumed they were on some kind of radio or something. Carman took the kids and me upstairs and showed me what to inventory and pack, and then plunged back into paperwork. Grant had to be on the next morning's plane, and they were taking no chances of his not making that flight. Carman would ship his things to him later.

Even with the time pressure and urgency, Al and Carman didn't lose their smiles for long. I was getting the feeling that foreign service officers had a code—maybe it was even written somewhere—that even if things are not okay, you *pretend* they are okay.

Carl was going to be shocked to find Grant gone—PNG'd. There'd been seven Americans on permanent status in this country. And now there were six.

I'd moved from place to place my entire life, both before and since we married, and I'd always been content. Equatorial Guinea would be a test, but I would make the best of it.

# 9

# RIO MUNI

*Carl was out* of communication when Grant was PNG'd for the same reason he would be unreachable the majority of the time. Most of his work was over on the mainland, in Rio Muni. Home to the Fang. He traveled throughout the interior with his team of vaccinators and his Fang–Spanish interpreter. I couldn't just pick up the phone and say, "Operator, connect me to the middle of the rainforest, please."

After Carl's initial face-off with the minister of health and the speedy approval of petrol for program vehicles, he expected to begin vaccinating in Rio Muni immediately. Macias first said four team members could fly to Bata, but he changed his mind. The fare, the equivalent of $8.57 per person, was too much. The team would have to travel overnight deck passage, $1.07, on the monthly sailing of the Spanish ship, the *Ciudad Toledo*. Carl adjusted his plan. He would get the program underway by mid July. But then President Macias insisted no one other than himself could sign for their boat tickets, which he did not do in time for a July 4 departure. This delayed departing for the mainland until the August 15 sailing.

During the delay, Carl moved offices. The State Department wasn't replacing Grant and offered the space to Carl.

Then, without the teams, he did an initial trial run of transportation details. (Not even his administrative assistant, Ricardo, was able to accompany him until *el presidente* approved those tickets.) At Bata, ships had to anchor a few hundred yards offshore, and the descent into the little motor launch was precarious, so Carl assessed how to deal with this for the vaccines and equipment. He'd heard how most of a shipload of grain and other commodities sent by Food for Peace sank to the bottom of the ocean as it was being off-loaded. The cargo was being stacked all along one side of the barge that would have ferried it to shore. The barge capsized and the cargo was lost. The smallpox program's shipments would be far smaller and not at risk for this kind of disaster.

The Spanish settled Rio Muni much later than they did the island, so the principal town, Bata, had far fewer amenities than our little town did. Besides the mainland presidential palace, Bata had a six-room hotel, a few cafés, a hospital and the notorious Bata Jail. It was also home to Radio Bata, which Carl used to announce vaccination sites and times.

Half the Rio Muni population lived in villages of fewer than two hundred people. Most of the Fang worked meager farms, often growing coffee. In the rain forest, tiny plots, a three- or four-foot irregular patch of level land wedged among the trees and their aboveground roots, constituted the farms and were watered by the continual mist. The men cleared the bits of land and worked cash crops. The women worked the food crops for the family and trekked to the nearest stream for water.

Polygamy was the rule rather than the exception. Children were considered part of the wealth of the family, so when a daughter married, her family was paid a dowry to compensate for the loss of childbearing potential as well as the loss of her labor.

Now that Macias had ordered all boats destroyed, hence no

fishermen, the Guineans' highly prized coastal fish was scarce. Salt-cured dried fish replaced fresh in the diet. Jungle crickets made excellent bait for stream fishing.

Carl saw chickens, goats, sheep and pigs in every village, but he said in his reports that they were rarely slaughtered. The people favored wild game (bushmeat). Favorites were monkey and hedgehog, but the meat of the local red-headed western lowland gorilla was sometimes on their tables as well.

In the interior of Rio Muni, many development programs had penetrated only as far as the roads could take them. Carl's teams had to reach everyone in the country, road or no road. The one tarred road along the coast and a cross-country road—from the coast to Macias's hometown on the Gabonese border—along with the more common unpaved roads had been adequate before independence. But the network was deteriorating. Our USAID trucks, with support equipment and kerosene-powered refrigerators for the vaccines, would go as far as possible, after which the Valiant motor scooters took the vaccinators deeper into the bush. Motorized canoes carried them up the streams that fingered their way to people living deep in the rainforest.

As with his destruction of all the boats on the coast and on the island, Macias had reportedly mined the main road leading out of Rio Muni and into Cameroon to prevent people leaving his country. Carl was mum on the topic of this widely circulated rumor.

A few months before our arrival, Macias's youth militia, in roaming gangs of up to a hundred, had terrorized people in the interior and murdered a Lebanese trader, triggering a general exodus of non-Africans. Among those who remained, Carl initially had three World Health Organization people—one a physician, one a sanitary engineer and the other an American nursing advisor—who could provide some pieces of information about the medical and political situations in their respective jurisdictions. Unfortunately, restrictions on where those people could go and what they could know significantly limited the scope of information they could provide, and all three left Equatorial Guinea during Carl's tour of duty.

Two foreigners, and only two, had letters from Macias allowing them to go anywhere in the country—an Australian mapping waterfalls around the world, and my husband. Aware of this special and no doubt tenuous access, he was circumspect in his information gathering. (From external sources, I've concluded Carl may have been gathering more information than just that related to smallpox and healthcare.)

Water supply failures as well as malfunctioning toilets and washing facilities plagued the hospitals in Rio Muni. And many older district hospitals had leaky roofs and no piped water at all. The facilities were understaffed and undersupplied for even the most rudimentary health services.

To make matters worse, the president micromanaged even the basic issue of supplies. Carl reported to CDC that when the Bata Hospital ran out of surgical gloves, they could not requisition more from the central dispensary on Fernando Po without the personal approval of President Macias.

Statistics on the number of hospitals and hospital beds were misleading because as foreigners exited, the handful of physicians dwindled. Many patients were seen by a *practicante*, a person who had received a brief paramedical training course that did not include nursing skills or techniques. Most people in these positions had finished secondary school, and a few had some experience working in a clinic. Even with such limited training, the practicantes had responsibilities much like interns in US teaching hospitals. They rotated call for nights, weekends and emergencies.

They diagnosed. They prescribed treatment. Some district hospitals and clinics had no MD, only a practicante, as the medical officer. Two districts had not even a practicante.

Students for healthcare training classes were most often chosen based on family or political relationships. Some of these had finished only primary school.

A few years later, all the trained and credentialed medical personnel would be gone, and healthcare would rest in the hands of Macias's family or those who had served him politically.

Despite these challenges few aid programs—by any country—were as well received by Macias and his xenophobic government. In the end, Carl was praised by our embassy for contributing to a more favorable US image in Equatorial Guinea.

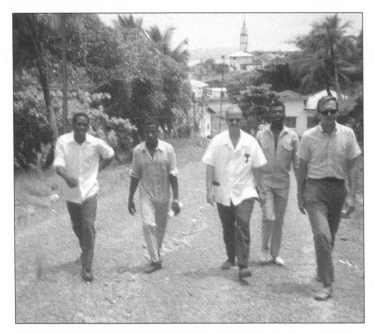

Carl and Dr. Martin Bradley with local smallpox team members

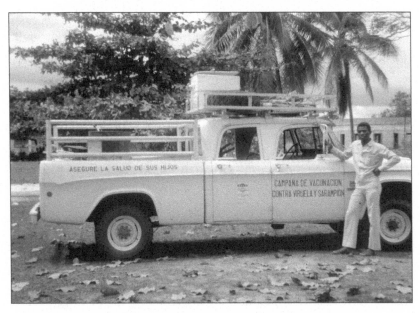

Team member with the smallpox truck

# 10

# NO TALKING TO LOCALS

*President Macias rigidly* enforced his decree against Equatorial Guineans entering the homes or offices of foreigners. In time, he even decreed that diplomats could talk to him and him only. They were forbidden to talk with any other locals.

The United Nations advisors could not advise because they were not allowed to talk to the locals whom they were there to assist and train. Just as with the UN expert in tropical agriculture who was never allowed to talk to his local counterpart or visit a farm, the decree precluded the very training and assistance that would allow an aid program to—well, provide aid. Fortunately for the worldwide war on smallpox, Chargé d'Affaires Al Williams met with Macias. Unbelievable as it sounds, he had to negotiate permission for Carl to talk to the vaccinators on his teams. (How Al managed any rapport with this cruel dictator mystified me, but he said his diplomatic mission would have accomplished nothing, absent an amicable relationship with the man running the country.)

Socially, Macias's edict had a demoralizing impact on all of us. We could socialize only with UN advisors, the sprinkling of Americans and Europeans who might come in for brief periods and personnel with embassies friendly to the United States. That gave us about twenty-five possible associates, most of whom were not English speaking.

Some UN advisors were reluctant to accept invitations from anyone connected with an embassy because the government recorded the names of all people entering their homes. Diplomats could not have a gathering of more than seven without special dispensation from Macias.

Months after our arrival, Macias's edict had too personal a consequence for us. Carl was working on the mainland for the week as usual, and I heard a scream from Charles's room in the middle of the night. I found him doubled over and clutching his abdomen, alternately moaning and screaming. Our night watchman knew where the doctor lived—about two blocks away.

I bundled my son into the truck. I knew Equatorial Guineans were forbidden to come to our house and we to theirs, but desperate for help—any at all—I hoped the doctor could come out to the truck and see Charles for a few moments. The watchman came back from the doctor's door with a message. "Please tell them I am very, very sorry, but I can't see him." The driver said the doctor looked terrified.

There were no foreign doctors to turn to, as Macias had driven them away. He had murdered or exiled most of his people who had more than an eighth-grade education and had expelled the nuns who worked with the hospital, so we wouldn't find even a nurse or a medical assistant of any kind. I had no way to phone Carl on the mainland. I could do nothing but return home, try to keep Charles comfortable and pray for the best. I had some Pepto Bismol and hoped that would help.

By 6:00 a.m. he was still in pain. I phoned the embassy residence. Not that they could help necessarily, but I hoped Al or Carman could think of something. I felt isolated. When Al arrived a few minutes later, we reviewed the facts and tried to come up with our nonmedical diagnosis. We concluded the problem was temporary and related to our picnic the day before with him and Carman. Charles had overindulged in the fresh coconuts scattered all over the beach, a novelty to us. I had no idea how the fresh oily coconut meat could pack into the gut. It would take a few hours for Charles to feel comfortable again, but at least we weren't dealing with appendicitis.

I learned that two Guinean doctors used to be here. One had been arrested at some point in the past few months, and the government gave out the story that, unfortunately, he died in prison. And the doctor I appealed to that night had just returned from exile. I hadn't realized foreigners could not even see the doctor without the president himself approving.

On this night, I felt as isolated as I've ever felt in my life.

Everything was less ominous in the daylight. But I now knew that in the event of a future medical emergency, we would need an airplane, not a truck.

# 11

## EVERYBODY COMES
## TO THE BAHIA

*Driving the quarter* mile down the curving spine of the harbor's
west arm, the bay to our right, we would pull up in front of Hotel
Bahia, perched on a promontory at the end of the finger of land.
The only hotel and indoor restaurant open to non-Africans, it was
an expat's most frequented destination on Fernando Po.

A bank of ten bare flag poles, one extending upward from
each letter of the sign HOTEL BAHIA, crested the upper floor
of an unremarkable white facade. Entering through the double
doors, we passed the reception desk and the stairway leading to
the sixteen guest rooms and walked through to the restaurant and
seaside tables beyond. The always-open wall of glass doors barely
separated indoor from outdoor dining.

Straight ahead, two tiny islets sat just yards off the shore, a
green semicolon. To the right the terrace stretched away toward
the harbor mouth, where a hundred feet below us the bay's placid
deep blue abruptly gave way to the soft gray ruffles of the open
sea. From there, one could also look back across the harbor to a
view of Santa Isabel's picturesque plaza.

On most days the sea disappeared into the mist of a slate-gray
distance. We'd gazed into that distance many times when one

crystal-clear day we saw it—the cone of West Africa's tallest and most active volcano. Mt. Cameroon soared its 13,255 feet out of the Atlantic only twenty miles away. We stood and drank in the view for a long time, because few days here would be so clear.

The Bahia's hands-on manager, Señor Careño, circulated through the restaurant or monitored things from behind the reception desk. I don't know when he first came to the island. I just know that after independence, Careño stayed on. After the government's barrage of fines and harassments, Careño stayed on. And after almost all other Spaniards chose to be evacuated, Careño stayed on.

And the wizened old gentleman at a corner table with only his brandy for company? His unkempt gray hair and sideburns and his heavy eyebrows framed eyes that stared blankly out to sea. Why had he stayed? Did he have nothing to go back to in Spain?

Few foreigners were brave enough—let's make that foolhardy enough—to come to the capital or the country these days, but the Hotel Bahia was home to those who did. And since it housed the one bar considered appropriate for expats and the town's one true restaurant, it was *the* place to go in Santa Isabel. It offered a much smaller, quieter, definitely tamer version of *Casablanca*'s "everybody comes to Rick's" kind of place, sans musicians. In the isolation and boredom of Macias's Equatorial Guinea, it was the place to find out who had been PNG'd this week. It was the place to watch and listen. A place filled with global political currents, international intrigue and furtive conversations in a hodge-podge of languages. It was the place to see the gradual flattening of expression in those who had stayed in this country too long or seen too much. And it was the place to have a delicious paella on Sundays.

The Bahia was the setting for the initial American diplomatic presence in the independent Republic of Equatorial Guinea. Al Williams told us the story. He'd been abruptly sent here from Senegal—told about the transfer the day after Christmas 1968, and had to leave Dakar on New Year's Eve night without benefit of a briefing and without Carman and the children. Equatorial Guinea had been independent not quite ninety days.

As his plane touched down in Santa Isabel, Al saw four DC-7s parked on the tarmac. They were white with huge red crosses painted on their sides. The relief flights of the ICRC (International Committee of the Red Cross) had been grounded.

Political pressure from Nigeria and from Britain, both of whom were eager for the Nigerian civil war to be over with Nigeria still intact, had grounded the relief flights for starving, blockaded Biafra. Al's mission, for which he did have a briefing, was to do everything he could to get those flights back in the air. His second mission was to establish a US embassy.

When he checked in at the Bahia, he found most of the rooms housed the brave Swiss or Swedish pilots and the support crews for the ICRC planes. The dangerous night flights into Biafra, with radio silence and landing lights flashed on only for a brief moment, flew food and relief supplies in and sometimes brought children out. Accusations abounded that these flights also brought weapons to the Biafrans. Unloading and reloading was quick and hazardous, often under fire.

Ambassador August Lindt, a Swiss diplomat and a member of the Lindt chocolate family, was head of the ICRC operation. He was Switzerland's ambassador to Moscow but was in Equatorial Guinea on loan, so to speak, to the relief operation.

Al told President Macias the eyes of the world were on Equatorial Guinea, and governments everywhere were perplexed as to why he had halted these humanitarian flights, which were only for the purpose of alleviating the suffering of Biafran women and children. His persuasiveness carried the day, and the planes were back in the air. By the end of the war on January 15, 1970, ICRC and two other agencies would estimate one million children had died during the Nigeria-Biafra conflict, and one million children were saved by the airlift. (Others would dispute these numbers and claim the Biafrans and sympathetic journalists had masterfully played the starvation card.)

Now Al could focus on opening an embassy. He had established his official residence in the oppressive heat of his second-floor room at the Bahia, where he laboriously coded and decoded cables. He had barely unpacked, he told us, when tensions reached crisis proportions between this infant republic and the eight thousand Spaniards who were still in the country. Neither side would yield an inch, especially not Spain's proud and severe Guardia Civil. Mobs and Equatorial Guinean soldiers eager to get their hands on liquor sacked the town's shops. Fear goaded the population. It was a powder keg.

On February 22, 1969, Macias's council of ministers created a paramilitary youth militia. They were called *Juventudes en Marcha con Macias*, "Youth on the March with Macias." Members were from his mainland Fang tribe, ages seven to thirty. Macias's inflammatory rhetoric incited the adolescent militia to molest Spaniards indiscriminately. Over in Rio Muni, gangs of a hundred roamed through the interior, intimidating non-Africans and conducting arbitrary searches of homes and shops. On Fernando Po, smaller gangs roamed the streets doing the same. The Spanish Guardia Civil retaliated with force. Macias declared a state of emergency, set a 6:00 p.m. to 6:00 a.m. curfew and used the Juventud to enforce it.

Al shared that, in the last week of February and the first week of March, Bahia's guests spent nervous nights during the standoff between locals and the Spaniards. Each evening about twenty Juventud members posted themselves at the door of the Bahia to make sure no one entered or departed. Al says they were "armed with clubs, bows and arrows and machetes" and were all "quite drunk with looted liquor." They pounced on any unsuspecting victim who happened to cross their path, beating them and robbing them of any money or jewelry.

Throughout the two weeks of curfew, dinner was served at the unheard of hour of 7:00 instead of at the customary 9:00 p.m. since electricity would be shut off at 8:00. On lockdown for the night, Al and the crews for the still-operating ICRC flights sat on the terrace, lit with candles kept on hand for the frequent power outages, sharing stories and, he says, "trying to drink enough Spanish brandy to sleep through the night."

During this standoff, Al asked US Consul Mike Hoyt in Douala, the man who'd been deep in conversation with Ambassador Hoffacker when we had come through the Douala airport, to come over for the weekend to assess the situation. In 1964, Mike and his key consular staff in Stanleyville, the Democratic Republic of the Congo (formerly the Belgian Congo), had been taken hostage and tortured by the Simbas. Belgian paratroopers rescued them 111 days later in a daring raid in which Simba machine guns mowed down hundreds of others.

Mike kept a daily log during captivity and would later write *Captive in the Congo*. He would also say on the record that the Stanleyville episode was no longer recognized by the State Department and was not included in their list of hostage situations or list of attacks against personnel.

Because of Mike's experience, Al wanted to know whether he thought the situation in Equatorial Guinea could deteriorate into a Congo-like scenario. He was "disheartened to hear that Mike considered it a distinct possibility."

Once Macias became president, he ordered the arrest of several of his country's leading political figures. Then came March 5, 1969, The Night of the Long Knives (according to foreigners) or "a date written in golden letters" (according to Macias). The president alleged his foreign minister, Ndongo Miyone, had attempted a coup, and the reprisals began. This happened fourteen months before we arrived. We'd learn more about it later.

More weeks of threats and maneuvers followed in the stand-off between Equatorial Guinea and Spain, and most Spaniards were ready to call it quits. Spain refused to withdraw its troops until its civilians were safely evacuated.

United Nations Secretary General U Thant sent his personal representative in March to prevent armed conflict between Guinean and Spanish forces and to negotiate a peaceful evacuation of Spanish civilians and their military after them. Under this protective shield, Spain amassed a conglomeration of passenger ships and cargo ships flying various national flags to evacuate its citizens. Al told us that four days of bedlam followed in the crowded harbor. The Spaniards had roots here, had lived here for decades. Now they swarmed onto the ships under a blanket of fear, with as many of their possessions as they could take with them.

From the Bahia's terrace, on April 4, 1969, Al watched a Spanish frigate lead eleven ships from the harbor single file, returning seven thousand people to Spain. The orderly line of ships slipped through the water and silently disappeared over the horizon.

Gone were all the technicians who ran the water works, the electrical plant, the hospital—all public services—and most of the teachers and medical personnel. Given that Macias was killing off all his own educated people, Al was watching the departure of all necessary skills for running the country, and the Spanish military's protection.

Few ships called at this inhospitable place after that.

—➔

Living in Macias's Equatorial Guinea, we needed laugh therapy. And lots of it. Al and Carman Williams were just the pair to provide it. They regaled us with the lighter side of the first year at this post. When Carman had finally been authorized to join Al, they rented an adjoining room to serve as a temporary chancery for meeting and entertaining visitors until they could lease and prepare a building. Al had arrived with necessary adornments for an embassy—including the American flag and the metal, two-foot-diameter Great Seal of the United States to be posted over the entrance. When serving guests in their hotel room/makeshift chancery, they used the Great Seal as a serving tray.

The stories that brought our biggest laugh, and still do, involved the then US ambassador to Equatorial Guinea, Albert "Bud" Sherer. He was also accredited to Togo, was resident there, and traveled to Santa Isabel for quarterly visits. (Later, State would combine the EG post with Cameroon rather than with Togo, due to its proximity.) During these visits, Sherer and Al had to make official calls on the president, cabinet ministers and government offices around town.

Enter the embassy car stories. Prior to the arrival of the black Chevy Nova as the official car, Al and Carman's Volkswagen Beetle served a tour of duty. It ran just fine—after a good push to get it started.

A graduate of Yale and Harvard Law, Ambassador Sherer was refinement personified. Al described Sherer as cultured, urbane, a man who had "arrived," as the saying goes. As they left each official visit in their best business suits and headed to the next, Al would say, "You steer, Mr. Ambassador, and I'll push," to which Ambassador Sherer always replied, "No. Carman will steer and we'll both push," which they did.

Then there's the afternoon Al and Ambassador Sherer drove down the coast to the one place where you could cool off in the Atlantic. They parked the VW, took off all but their swim trunks, and left their clothes in the car. While they were at the beach, their clothes were stolen. America's two highest-level representatives to this country walked the few miles back to town, bare-chested, wearing only swim trunks and carrying towels. The keys to the recalcitrant car had been in a pants pocket.

Seven months after Al first arrived at this post, he and Carman left the Bahia, moved themselves into an official residence and the office into its official chancery home, complete with steel vault. On July 24, 1969, they held a reception to celebrate the opening, which would become official on August 1.

We spent many hours with Al and Carman at the Bahia, at the residence or in our home. They shared stories, some funny, some frightening—much of which could be overheard by our children. If only I had known then what Mike and Jo Hoyt had learned when their three-year-old son resisted boarding the little plane evacuating him and his mother out of Stanleyville. He wailed, "Will they throw me out of the airplane when we land?" Recounting this in his book, Mike says that a few weeks earlier the boy had been playing in the living room while the adults socialized, and he must have heard them talking about the assassination of Patrice Lumumba.

At the Bahia, eccentricity often seemed a prerequisite. Some diplomat or adventurer always had a bizarre but true story, often accompanied by the latest whispered news. The escapism could almost lull us into forgetting where we were. Consigned to our insular life, we ignored the time. But eventually we had to leave the Bahia and walk or drive home through silent streets.

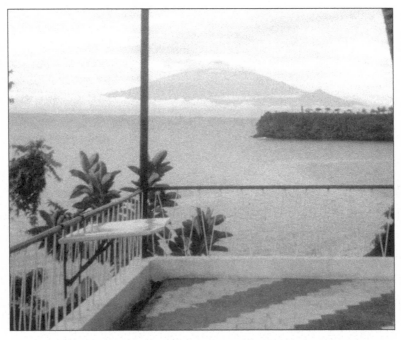

Rare view of Mt. Cameroon from Hotel Bahia's terrace

# 12

## MACIAS NGUEMA

*These streets hadn't* always been so deserted. On October 12, 1968, the plaza and the town were packed and pulsing. Dancing and singing, parades and speeches hailed the end of colonial rule. The people were independent. They had a constitution. They themselves had chosen a president. They had one of the highest per capita incomes in Africa. They numbered doctors, teachers and technicians among their citizenry. The future was bright.

How had a year silenced a city? How were uncles and brothers disappearing—or reappearing with vacant faces and mangled bodies? How had education become a crime punishable by torture? How were basic services plummeting toward nonexistence? Mystery as impenetrable as the rain forest shrouded much. But Al and Carman and our UN friends filled us in on what they knew. I would have to learn the rest with later research.

When Spain sponsored the first election the month before independence, few expected Francisco Macias Nguema to win. The other three candidates were more popular and better educated. Most observers dismissed poorly educated, sleepy-eyed Macias as a "backwoodsman."

But he was cunning. He shrewdly hid his lack of education by promising a return to Fang tribal practices and traditions.

He despised "intellectuals," his term for the educated. Bitterly anti-Spanish, some said rabidly so, he ran on a platform of ridding the country of every vestige of colonial rule. He drew in the crowds with his emotional rhetoric and promised that once he got rid of all the colonialists, people would have endless prosperity. Everything would be great.

He bested Bonifacio Ondo Edu in a runoff election. Francisco Macias Nguema became president, and Ondo Edu disappeared. Al could find out nothing about what had happened to Edu. People who might have known something were too frightened to talk. It was later learned he had taken refuge in Gabon as soon as Macias won the election.

On March 5, 1969, a date "written in golden letters" (a phrase Macias used time and again as a rallying cry), Macias announced that his foreign minister, Ndongo Miyone, had attempted to overthrow him in a coup and then committed suicide. There would be several different versions of how Ndongo met his end, but Macias, who during the standoff with the Spanish had left the island to spend time in his mainland palace in Bata, summoned Chargé d'Affaires Williams to Bata, where he rolled out his version.

Al told us he was cooling off in the little pool at the Bahia when he received a telegram.

COME TO BATA STOP I HAVE SOMETHING TO TAKE UP
WITH YOU STOP PRESIDENT MACIAS STOP

To say that Al was apprehensive as he flew to Bata may be an understatement. When he arrived at the palace, Macias motioned for Al to follow him upstairs. He then showed Al a bedroom and adjoining bathroom, saying Ndongo had barricaded himself in this room when loyalist troops cornered him. Then with apparent satisfaction, Macias showed Al the bathroom window from which he claimed Ndongo had jumped to his death onto the concrete patio below.

Whether real, imagined or fabricated, the coup was the excuse to launch what would become known as "The Terror." Macias added Ndongo's title to his own. He was now head of the foreign ministry as well as president. Equatorial Guinea, this sad little infant country, was barely six months old.

In The Terror's opening salvo, Macias had Ondo Edu extradited on trumped-up charges and soon executed him. Next to be murdered were the other contenders in the presidential campaign, then traditional clan chiefs and those who had led the independence movement—anyone viewed as a leader—and the wives or other relatives of these people.

Just as Franco's Spain, itself no example of democratic government, had left its former colony ill-prepared for independence, Spain was ill-prepared for a ruthless, vindictive killer in the presidential palace, their former governor general's mansion.

But Macias Nguema had been fooling the Spanish for years, not a hard thing to do since Spain paid scant attention to the mainland, Rio Muni. Had they bothered to acquaint themselves with the Fang or their language, they might have seen this man's long record of corruption and cruelty and not facilitated his political advancement.

Macias was the son of a revered witchdoctor in the Esangui, a subgroup of one of the fifty Fang clans, in the town of Mongomo on Rio Muni's eastern border with Gabon. They believed the elder Nguema, reportedly a leader in the Bwiti cult, had great powers. They called him *Su Santo Padre*, "His Saintly Father."

Macias Nguema's year and place of birth are disputed, and little is known of his early life. The few fragments of information point to his having grown up in a violent environment, with witchcraft a prominent presence. Some say Macias's father forced young Macias to watch as he killed Macias's little brother in a witchcraft ceremony. This and other variations on the story are unverified due to the secret nature of the Bwiti.

It is known Macias did poorly in secondary school and failed the civil service entrance examination three times. After passing on the fourth try, he held a series of low-level jobs in the colonial bureaucracy. What he lacked in education he made up for with trickery. He slyly promoted himself, especially in his job as Fang–Spanish interpreter in the court in Mongomo.

With the Spaniards' ignorance of the local language, Macias could twist the facts and interpret for or against people as he chose. He warned minor offenders they would be handed harsh sentences but claimed he could use his influence to get their sentences reduced—for the right price. If he received a large enough bribe, he interpreted in a way that would bring a favorable court ruling. If not, he could bring disaster down on the accused. Neither the Spanish nor the accused were the wiser.

What the Spanish did notice was the influence Macias appeared to have among the people, so they installed him as *alcalde* (mayor) of Mongomo. Despite privately detesting the Spanish, he never placed himself in any position Spain opposed, so the colonialists assumed that here was a man who would do their bidding. They awarded him the Order of Africa and continued to give him more promotions.

When Spain set up an "autonomous government" (1964–1968), allowing locals to have a say in their domestic affairs, it installed Macias as minister of public works and deputy president. Ondo Edu, also a Fang, was president. Macias's unexplained rapid promotions, from assistant interpreter to mayor to deputy president, all in one year, did not lessen his hatred of the Spanish—or of anyone in authority over him.

The 1967 conference Spain convened to draft a constitution

included more than forty Guineans and more than twenty Spaniards. Macias's speeches at the conference have been characterized as incoherent fury. And they were reportedly full of numerous appeals to the chairman to let him finish. One commentator said the speeches defied analysis of his political thought and "what Macias wanted may not have been very clear, but it was evident that he wanted it very strongly." A sample text of one of these incoherent rants includes his assertion, "I consider Hitler to be the savior of Africa."

Macias had a talent for stirring the crowds despite his lack of coherent speech and lack of a program. In the presidential race, the upset victory was due to that skill, and to the backing of one Spanish law professor who groomed him, funded a glossy advertising campaign, managed campaign strategy and took over the speech-writing, thinking he would control Macias to his own advantage.

A large percentage of the people who were drawn to the impassioned oratory of Macias didn't know what a vote was for—any vote. And, as someone later observed, now they would never need to know.

One Guinean explained that votes are cast first for family members and then clan members above all others, no matter how bad the candidate. He said the country is the last thing an African considers. But Uncle Macias had long demonstrated his sly cruelty in his hometown. He lost in Mongomo.

Before our family arrived in Santa Isabel, Macias had finished killing off his obvious political opponents and wives of those men, and he now targeted doctors, teachers, civil servants—anyone with education or specialized technical training. They were intellectuals and therefore a threat to his personal control. The educated Bubis and Fernandinos caught the initial brunt of his fury, and most were dead or had fled before we stepped onto the tarmac in Santa Isabel. Most of those who remained resorted to silence for survival.

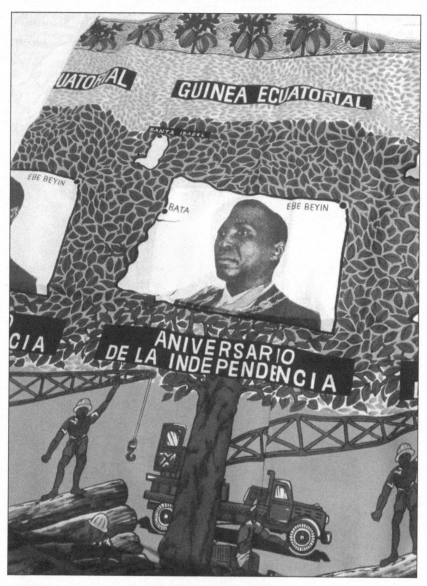

Fabric with image of Macias

# 13

## NOT A GAME

*The damp dress* clung to my skin in the sticky equatorial heat. I plucked fabric away from my body and hoped walking would create airflow. I was focused on that futile effort and on my grocery list when a man coming around the next corner stopped dead in his tracks. A woman across the street from him froze midstride. Then the only other person on the street, a man a little closer to me, did the same. Like a childhood game of "statue." I didn't move a muscle.

El presidente had once again gotten a whim to raise or lower the flag over the presidential palace. It could happen anytime, day or night, and no one dare defy his latest fiat. Someone near the palace had heard the signal over the loudspeaker. The statue effect then proceeded away from the palace from person to person, like ripples from a pebble tossed into a pond. Not being within sight or earshot of the palace did not relieve one of responsibility or protect one from punishment. You could always see a person at the next corner or down the street who froze midstep. And you'd better do likewise.

The consequence of noncompliance, at least for the country's citizens and for some particularly disliked foreigners, would be determined at the time of infraction. And it would depend on the enforcer's mood of the moment.

Macias used three groups to terrorize his people. From what I heard of the three, I thought a person would hope for the police. A policeman on Fernando Po might only kick you or slap you around if you were lucky. Or you could wind up in the jail at the police station.

Next most severe might be one—or a gang—of the Juventude. We were told these kids would be in plain clothes but armed, and would likely take any money, jewelry or other property for personal use before beating you up with a club. It was said that when they wanted money, they just made a cash withdrawal from anyone unfortunate enough to be in their path.

The most dreaded enforcer would be one of Macias's usually drunk Guardia Nacional. When one of the Guardia enforced some edict, he leaned more toward beating you to a pulp with a rifle butt and then handcuffing and dragging you off to Black Beach Prison.

I never witnessed any of these things, but I didn't need to see to be convinced. I remained frozen in position until the gentleman farthest from me in the direction of the palace resumed walking. As I continued on to the grocer's, the other two people whose actions had provided my signal walked past me, eyes turned away. They would not risk being accused of contact with a foreigner.

I exhaled—and walked on down the near-empty and silent street toward the store.

---

Decades later I would learn of Charles's fear that we would be shot during one of these "statue" episodes, that as I gripped Ginger's hand or held her she would squirm or wiggle and we would all be killed. What did he overhear in our home or in the embassy? What did his playmates tell him of their own families' suffering at the hands of Macias?

## Reflection

no bells, no horns
no shouts of hawkers
silence
beautiful, silent, cover of murder
like a marble mausoleum
beautiful, silent, cover of death

in Official American cocoon
safe, I walk quiet streets
walking through mausoleum
torture and killing just out of sight

I don't hear the screams

# 14

## SAMUEL'S DOMAIN

*Despite the tragedy* and the drama of this place, there was a comforting everydayness to life inside the house. Carl had found a gem when he hired Samuel. (At work he found another real gem in his administrative assistant, Ricardo, on whom he relied heavily.)

Our whole family formed a real attachment to Samuel and he to us. This man with such a warm and gentle spirit had left his family behind in Nigeria for better wages on Fernando Po.

One day I got out our World Atlas. I first pointed out Nigeria on a world map. Then I narrowed the focus. From a map of the appropriate hemisphere, I paged to the African continent and finally to the map of Nigeria. I asked Samuel the name of the town nearest his home village and then pointed to its name on the map, along with the river where he swam as a little boy.

"Oh, madame, how do men know these things? Are they gods?" In these days before satellites, I didn't fully understand how map details could be determined either, but I was glad I could share those details with this good man and good friend.

Samuel worked in our home five days a week. Three others worked part time, all Igbo from eastern Nigeria. Blessing, our laundry man, came two times a week. Two young men, in their twenties I'd guess, were employees of the embassy and did odd jobs for us now and then. Their names were Sunday and Friday. Many Africans were named for the day on which they were born.

I would cook more here than I had in Kano. I had plenty of time. No princesses to visit. No Sarki Trader. Carl on the mainland most of the time. I continued to practice my curry and samosas. My brass mortar and pestle were kept busy pulverizing the dozen or so spices for the curry. Fenugreek seeds and whole cloves weren't easy to grind into powder.

The local diet consisted primarily of plantains, manioc (a starchy tuber also known as cassava or yucca) and dried fish, so besides plantains and the papayas and bananas from our yard, I relied on my commissary orders of canned foods—tuna fish, Spam (yes, Spam), green beans and spinach, along with grains and powdered milk. When Samuel went to shop for an item at the grocery store on occasion, he commonly returned with the news, "Sorry, madame. It's finish." A couple of times a month, fresh meat arrived from Cameroon. Each customer was allowed two kilos. Frozen beef and chicken arrived once a month from Spain, but those would sell out in the first week. Thanks to our big deep freeze for the vaccine, we ordered thirty frozen chickens each month. I learned to prepare chicken in every way known to woman—stove top, since our oven didn't work. I tried out new recipes for cold buffets, such as salmon mousse and cauliflower "frosted" with avocado puree. New culinary adventures separated me from the realities hiding just outside the door.

As in Kano, we boiled and filtered all water. Carl said we'd have to plan for gaps in the water supply by storing extra in large cans. In the dry season, we had no water between 1:00 and 4:00 p.m. and between 9:00 p.m. and 6:00 a.m. That beautiful bay and the other waters around the island were so picture perfect I seldom thought about the fact that all the sewage, raw sewage, was dumped into them.

On one of the days I was out, Charles set a fire in our backyard—near the generator. Samuel rushed buckets of water from the kitchen to put it out. Thank goodness the fire wasn't set between 1:00 and 4:00 p.m.

We had been advised to bring plenty of batteries and lightbulbs, but with the many power outages our bulbs would have little likelihood of needing replacement.

Charles and Ginger were young enough to share a bedroom for now, and a "cold room" was important. We could keep that room's evaporative cooler at its coldest setting to protect film, cameras, tools, leather sandals—anything that could rot, rust or disintegrate.

And that deep freeze—I didn't like having it in the hallway. I wanted to move the freezer into our cold room before we started filling it. (I was big on painting or rearranging furniture when Carl was away.) One afternoon I set to work. I measured and figured I could push the deep freeze through the bedroom door if those big hinges weren't in the way. No problem. I would just unscrew the hinges where they attached to the chest, lift the lid off, and reattach it once I had the chest where I wanted it.

On my knees behind the freezer, making progress on loosening the last screw, I gave no thought to the powerful spring that allows these lids to open with the slightest one-finger lift. The screw's release set free the giant hinge. It hit my forehead with such force it knocked me out—for a second? A minute? I'm not sure. To this day, the inch-long dent front and center in my skull is a reminder to use more common sense. I'm sure Samuel was off that day or he would have prevented my foolish mistake.

# 15

# BROTHER TO BROTHER

*In mid June* 1970, six weeks after his arrival in Santa Isabel, Carl wrote the following letter to his brother, sharing some of the more unusual Equatorial Guinea happenings.

Dear Ken,

The new assignment is really interesting and certainly different from Kano. Under Equatorial Guinea's dictator, the place is a political funny farm and to even start a discussion of that would take at least a day or so. Enclosed is a publication on E. G. from the State Dept. Published in April, 1969. Since the alleged coup d'etat in 1969, things have gone downhill for the foreign community here to say nothing of the day-by-day hell the local people have to endure. And the hatred for the Spanish here is something you wouldn't believe.

Everywhere you go there are police and the Guardia Nacional with weapons. Coming into the Santa Isabel airport, everyone except those of us with Diplomatic or Official status wind up in a back room for a complete physical and personal baggage search under rifle. Everywhere we go the police who are watching us write down when we left, and when we get to where we're going, the police at that location write down when we arrived.

Everyone is open to suspicion. A few weeks ago our third officer in the Embassy was declared persona non grata (PNG) and given 24 hours to get out of the country. PNG is a way of operating around here on the part of the immature xenophobic government hated by most of its neighbors and, I believe, by most of its people.

The Nigerian laborers are treated like dogs and now that the war is over in Nigeria they're starting to go home. The whole economy of this place is going to pot because the Guineans have gotten used to the Nigerians doing all the work. It must be an escape from the hopelessness of living under this brutal government, but many are replacing meals with booze.

Fortunately, all of us appear to be in the same boat around here. The Russians up the street ½ a block away keep themselves locked up. The Nigerian Embassy and its staff have had hard times recently. There are five or six North Koreans running around here raising hell and trying to get recognition from the government, but to date they haven't been recognized. The Spanish ambassador is always under suspicion. Now that he has just married an American girl who will arrive next week, I'm sure over in the Presidential Palace they'll be saying the Spanish and the Americans are in a joint plot to overthrow the government.

Since the publication of the April '69 booklet I'm sending you, the whole section on the political conditions, economy, foreign relations and US-EG relations have changed, and not for the better. It's a national and human tragedy that makes one appreciate very dearly the freedoms under law we have as Americans. We have problems, of course, but when one looks at the suspension of human freedoms by an irrational government one realizes we're not as bad as some would have you believe.

There is humor in all of this too. Like the North Koreans hanging anti-American propaganda calendars around town and our chargé d'affaires going around taking them down. Etc. Etc.

One could go on and on. All in all, our safety is guaranteed here by the United States as much as anyone's safety can be guaranteed in the world today, especially in this neck of the woods.

You'd never believe the physical beauty of this place. I hope the enclosed booklet will give you some idea. Last Friday night Charles and I took the Spanish ship overnight from Santa Isabel to Bata. That was great fun.

Finally, Ken, please don't leave this letter lying around as you never know who'll get hold of it. I trust you'll understand.

Take good care of yourself, Bro,
Carl

———

Carl bragged on Charles's bravery in what to me would be a harrowing descent down the rope ladder from the ship to the tiny target below, the tender to take them to the beach. There was no pier. I assume Carl had to hold him going down the ladder, as the rungs would be too far apart for five-year-old legs. Charles doesn't remember the descent or much about the boat, but he has a snippet of memory of being in a jungle and his dad hacking at undergrowth with a machete.

# 16

## THE SHIPMENT

*Soon after daylight* I opened our louvered shutters, their varnish always sticky in this half mile between sea and rain forest. Carl grinned as we pushed the State Department furniture against the walls. It was summer here near the equator, but today would be like Christmas and birthdays rolled into one. After a full year of crawling from port to port between Santa Fe and Santa Isabel, our missing household shipment was arriving. Nothing could spoil this day, June 19, 1970.

New books, crafts and educational toys would enhance these TV-free years I so cherished. Many of the children's clothes and shoes I'd bought to cover two years of projected growth would be outgrown, but I hoped at least half would still fit. We'd follow our usual plan for a move into a new place—put things in order as we unpacked.

Charles, now five, ran back and forth through the house but stopped now and then to make more room for the arrival of re-membered favorites, especially his jumbo cardboard building blocks. Ginger stayed in an out-of-the-way corner, lost in an imaginary world with her baby dolls.

Carl jumped in his truck and headed to the airport. He and Chargé d'Affaires Al Williams would meet the monthly Pan

African Airlines support flight bringing its routine shipment of embassy supplies and commissary orders along with our sea shipment.

I rearranged kitchen shelves to make room for pots and pans, spices and cookbooks.

Charles stopped running and stood watch at the front window. With his excited, "It's here!" I started out the door. Then stopped cold. Carl bolted from his truck and slammed the door. Right behind him, a bunch of Guardia Nacional piled out of their Land Rover. Carl's eyes could have set a bonfire ablaze as he stomped past me into the house with the first box.

He hissed through clenched teeth. "These guys showed up at the airport before the flight landed. They're gonna search every bit of our shipment. I wanted Al to ask the comandante to *at least* limit the number of Guardia in our house. You know what he told me? He said they are 'perfectly within their rights to do just what they want to do!' But I won't stand for this!"

I put my hand on Carl's arm. I knew my words would accomplish nothing. But then, neither did my gesture. Samuel had arrived, and I asked him to take Charles and Ginger to their room. Ginger easily returned to her private mental and physical space, but Charles kept watch, peering from behind his door as Carl and Samuel carried things into the house.

Several boxes were still in the yard and on our postage stamp–size porch when Carl had to rush back to the airport where Al and the comandante waited with the rest of the shipment. He had no choice but to leave us alone with some of the Guardia—maybe four? Surely it was more. They stood guard over the boxes in the yard.

Soon after Carl left, it started raining. I determined to keep at least some boxes dry, especially ones labeled *Books*. I carried one inside over the objection of one of the Guardia. He started to follow me into the house and wanted to search that box plus the ones already inside.

I told him in Spanish he'd have to wait until my husband and the chargé d'affaires arrived. He shouted something at me I didn't understand. I put on a brave front—and it was a front—and repeated the same message:

*"No. Por favor. Tiene que esperar a mi esposo y el encargado de negocios."*

The Guardia were not used to being told no and didn't tolerate being crossed. I could have done nothing had he tried to force his way into the house. Thankfully, he just stationed himself in front of our door, his arms barring entry or exit. It hadn't taken long here in Equatorial Guinea for us to learn that the Guardia's actions were erratic, so I wasn't about to attempt to cross that barrier. Some of our shipment would be lost to the rain. I locked the door and waited.

It felt like hours—might have been one—before Carl and Al, the rest of the shipment, and the comandante arrived—with more Guardia. Despite protests from Carl and me, seven Guardia crowded into our living room with their semiautomatic rifles and fixed bayonets.

The comandante ordered everyone into our front room, but we had Samuel keep Charles and Ginger off to one side as much as possible. Al stayed back in the connecting dining room. When all were assembled, the comandante signaled us to unpack.

Carl and I sat on the floor facing each other, our boxes between us. The seven soldiers surrounded us. Carl and I each chose a box. The Guardia held seven rifles poised and aimed at the boxes we had chosen.

I slit the tape on my first box, opened the flaps—and *thwack!* The tip and rusty shaft of the first bayonet disappeared into a box full of toddler shoes and pajamas. Two other Guardia followed suit. *Thwack! Thwack!* What were we trying to smuggle under those toddler clothes?

Next box. *Thwack!* The bayonets hit our picture albums, piercing holes in old family photos. Next box. Light bulbs splintered. Defenseless.

Carl's boxes got the same treatment.

The Guardia were especially aggressive against any item that could conceal something else.

Tupperware containers with lids to keep bad things out and good things in were among the suspects. Now full of bayonet holes, they'd serve as strainers.

Then Carl's toolbox. Where had Carl put that key when we packed up a year ago? Where was that key? Neither of us could think, and pressure was mounting. The bayonet wielders grew impatient. Finally, one of the Guardia swung down hard with the butt of his rifle and broke the box wide open.

Our commissary order had arrived on the same flight as our household shipment. The Guardia pierced and tore open not just cases but individual packets. Beans, macaroni, powdered milk and grains of rice covered the floor.

*Is Charles wondering why mom and dad aren't stopping the bad guys, or if a Guardia will stab him with a bayonet? What's Ginger thinking?*

Little things, tiny things, gripped my attention. The Guardia's rumpled and stained dark green fatigues formed a blurred backdrop for the dirty finger on the trigger of the rifle two feet away. The light glinting off a shiny spot on the bayonet grabbed me more than the acrid smell of liquored and sweaty bodies in our tight, sweltering space.

Rifles swung around, unpredictable and uncontrolled. *A rifle is going to go off any minute . . . some of these guys are pretty soused.*

The Guardia launched preemptive bayonet strikes into

Charles's cardboard building blocks. The scene played out in jerky, disjointed frames like an old silent movie reel. Was this reality or a nightmare?

*Just keep quiet, Bee . . . don't startle these guys . . . no sudden moves.*
Okay. Next box.
*Breathe, Bee. Okay. Breathe. Just breathe.*

Charles saw me open a box of his toys and was trying for a closer look. One of the Guardia planted his rifle butt on the floor next to him. The length of his rifle pressed against his arm and shoulder. I arrested my reflexive reaction to grab it.

Seeing the rifle shoved against Charles, Carl arrived at full-on tooth-grinding-about-to-explode mode.

At that instant, Al stepped in. *Well, finally. It's about time!* With a conspiratorial smile and buttery voice, he approached the comandante. The two of them left the room for a few moments. When they returned, Al had negotiated permission for Samuel to take Charles and Ginger and a few toys to the backyard. He must have convinced the comandante their job would be far easier with no children underfoot.

Al tried to further calm the gathering storm. He steered me out the back door in the direction of the papaya and banana trees. "Bee, there's no need to worry. It's all just—"

Carl stormed out close behind, his jaw set. Never concerned about his personal safety, he fumed.

"Al, I won't tolerate this risk to Bee and the kids."

"If we're calm—"

"You've got to put a stop—"

"We could make it more dangerous if we—"

My husband stiffened as Al put a hand on his shoulder.

"The ambassador will hear about this!"

"You have to chalk it up to representation, Carl."

I decided the phrase must be scripted in a foreign service

officer's handbook somewhere. A diplomat's response in crisis: representation. I had thought this foreign service lingo just referred to diplomatic dinners and parties paid for with a representation budget. I was wrong.

On the patio, Ginger rocked on the rocking horse Grandpa had made. Charles had been listening to the adults and chewing on his fingers. Now Samuel called to him, and he started playing with his newly arrived fire engine.

As Al, Carl and I headed back toward the house, Carl put his arm around me. His muscles were taut and his fingers dug into my upper arm. His rapid breathing seemed deafening as we followed the chargé d'affaires back inside. But he clamped his lips and didn't say a word. The stakes were too high.

*Pull yourself together, Bee. The kids are safe now. Have to finish* "representing the United States of America."

Grips on the rifles loosened, and bodies slouched as the hours crawled into afternoon. The temperature and humidity rose in our living room. We offered cold drinks.

By the time the Guardia stabbed the last box, numbness deadened my remaining nerve fragments. Carl seethed again as Al actually thanked the comandante for his service. Later we would realize the professional diplomat knew his business and had taken the least dangerous course. But in the moment, I was puzzled, tense, and Carl was furious. I had yet to learn that to the diplomat, representation very often means being in harm's way and putting the best face on it.

Despite my vivid memory of much of that day, for some reason I cannot recall the Guardia's leaving, although I know they departed.

Ginger remembers only what she saw at her two-year-old eye-level. Boxes and legs—and a flash of bayonets that held no meaning for her. A change in Charles's play after the event had given me at least a partial answer as to what he'd felt. Since the first moon landing the previous year, much of his play had been in the cardboard-and-aluminum-foil lunar lander he'd made. After his brush with the Guardia, his creation with the bayonet-riddled blocks was a fortress which he defended with his handmade swords. He recruited his chalkboard as a functioning drawbridge over a moat.

—➤

The day after the invasive experience, Carl wrote a detailed account to CDC. His last paragraph said:

> The following questions have to be asked, and I would hope answered, in light of these events: . . . What protection do we in fact have in this assignment? . . . As I will be separated from my family much of the time in the coming months, and as my communications and movements will be strictly at the discretion of the Government of Equatorial Guinea once I leave the island, I expect . . . a reasonable guarantee of protection for my family.

He protested that representing America shouldn't necessitate endangering our children and me. He added, "There will not be any compromise on my part in regard to my family's safety and well-being."

I'll find a place to keep that memo. Maybe in the photo albums with their stab wounds from the Guardia.

# 17

# THE SPANISH AMBASSADOR'S BRIDE

*Journal note: June 22, 1970*

Oh my goodness! This place is in such a dither. Our little expat community has never been so excited. This week the Spanish ambassador, Ambassador Manolo Garcia Miranda, arrives back from home leave—and honeymoon! Any new arrival excites our tiny enclave. With this we'll get a huge shot in the arm. He's bringing his new bride!

*Journal note: June 27, 1970*

Wow! We've gone beyond excitement here. A reception to welcome Barbara set off social fireworks. I'd guess she's at least thirty or even thirty-five years younger than the ambassador. She's statuesque—blond—and American! Garcia Miranda met Barbara in New York at the UN headquarters where she worked as an interpreter. She seems very friendly. Even though she's the Spanish ambassador's wife, it's nice to have a third American woman in the country. Yay.

I get the feeling Barbara will be the hostess with the mostest. Great to have something going on here besides the grim and gruesome—for a change. And lots to talk about!

One work-related note: three days ago the National Communicable Disease Center changed its name to the Center for Disease Control. We've almost always just said CDC anyway. Now we can officially drop the N.

# 18

# TUMBU FLY

*A traumatic event* involving the tumbu fly prompted this letter.

Well, dear ones, today I fired our laundry man. His name is Blessing, but I'm afraid that in our employ he hasn't quite lived up to his name. You may be shocked I could fire anyone, but I claim just cause. Sometimes in the rainy season, it rains three days and nights without pause—pours in buckets! And I mean pours. When we get a break in the weather, we race to get the wet clothes hung on the line, hoping they can at least partially dry in this hot moist air before the next rain.

Drum roll here for the attack—of—the—TUM-bu flies. They lay their eggs on damp laundry as it's "drying." If sheets and clothes aren't ironed thoroughly enough to kill the eggs, they attach themselves to a person's flesh, burrow in, and morph into larvae, which grow into big creepy mounds under the skin! You can see them moving around under there—ick!

Blessing has been slack in his ironing performance, barely warming the clothes, much less getting them hot enough to kill those tumbu eggs, and I've given him

several warnings. Today I discovered three of these larvae in an area around Ginger's ribcage. I can't say forcing
them out hurt me worse than it hurt her, but it was a close
second, and it nearly killed Carl when I told him about
it. Poor Ginger. That did it. Blessing will now be blessing
some other family.

Of course, this wet climate has its beneficial aspects.
A few months ago I broke a limb off our papaya tree and
just stuck it in the ground a few feet away. In about a week
there were tiny shoots of a new tree, and before long we'll
enjoy even more papayas. Besides the delicious fruit, we'll
have plenty of leaves to wrap around cuts of meat that
need tenderizing.

In other weather-related news, we use plastic containers to protect cameras, batteries, film, and photos—and
keep them in our cold room. But we didn't know our
books would be at risk. We've just discovered even the
tiniest of little critters can have a hunger for knowledge—
love munching their way through moistened binding
glue, that is. Over half our books, Carl's beloved history
books and my speech pathology texts included, are about
to fall apart, so we've now moved them into the cold room
as well. We store postage stamps and tape in plastic bags
to protect the glue. Locally purchased envelopes have no
glue.

That reminds me, they're about to close the diplomatic
pouch and I want this letter to be in it, so I'll have to say
bye for now. Gotta fetch the tape to seal the envelope, and
hope that when I lick the stamp it still has glue. Please
write soon!

# 19

# FOURTH OF JULY

*My Independence Day note:*

If you've ever celebrated July Fourth in a country with a complete lack of liberty, you've had a glimpse of how emotional we were last night. The American chargé d'affaires and his wife hosted a dinner for our tiny handful of Americans and a few guests from the diplomatic corps.

It just so happened this month's movie was *The Comedians*, based on Graham Greene's novel of the same name. What an eerie experience to watch it—here! If you read the book or watch the movie, you'll have an idea of what it's like in Equatorial Guinea.

Before we adjourned, the chargé played a recording of the "Star Spangled Banner," and we Americans stood there, hands over hearts, tears streaming down our oh-so-solemn faces. I have never been as stirred by the anthem as I was last night.

Enjoy your summer in the Land of the Free.

*The Flip Side of Freedom:*

Macias had his own July celebration, the formation of the single political party. He said in a rousing speech (at least the English translation looks rousing) on July 7, that Guineans had "made evident the need for national unity by the creation of a single Party." He said the existence of various political parties on the eve of independence was a "confused situation . . . [that] confronted us with difficulties of enormous profundity."

I include here excerpts of the official printed English translation of Macias's speech—including the capital letters and all punctuation. Item seven from the official act proclaimed their "collective desire for the TOTAL ABOLITION of those pre-independence political Movements and Parties and the subsequent creation of a SINGLE POLITICAL PARTY," the Partido Unico Nacional (PUN), "from henceforth the only legal Party of our nation." He ended his speech saying, "No honest Guinean worthy of that name can live outside that decisive action that binds us to the P.U.N. This is a date on which we have chosen a new way . . . LONG LIVE THE P.U.N.!!!"

Rumors are that besides abolishing all other parties, the Juventudes en Marcha con Macias is perhaps being beefed up. They're given military training, these seven- to thirty-year-olds.

# 20

# EMBASSY COMIC RELIEF

*"Could we just* have a hot dog this time? Please?"

Ginger or Charles begging for hot dogs? No. The Spanish ambassador's American bride, Barbara Garcia Miranda. She was coming to our house for lunch again tomorrow and wanted to preempt my menu planning with her emergency request. She said she just had to escape all the formality once in a while and was homesick for an American hot dog.

"Your wish is my command, Barbara. Commissary order to the rescue. A little Spam on the side?"

"Ha! Very funny, Bee."

Three American women lived on Fernando Po now. I hoped Ambassador Garcia Miranda had been upfront with Barbara about what her life might be like in Equatorial Guinea. When she and I were together, we stayed away from the topic.

On the social side, Barbara had quickly risen to the challenge of putting on elegant events at the Spanish embassy. Less than a month after her arrival, she hosted her first official event, the *Fiesta Nacional de España*. The invitation to a noon reception on July 18 bore the customary address, to Señor Don Carl Bloeser y Señora.

Before long Barbara and Ambassador Garcia Miranda's calendar was full of lively dinners. I'd tell her I didn't know how she did it. And she'd tell me I could do it too if I had all the staff she had.

The embassy's massive mahogany banquet table, polished so it could pass for a mirror, seated about twenty-four to the best of my memory. Six- or seven-course dinners for every friendly diplomat, any aid worker in town and any visiting businessmen, along with Careño from the Bahia, were escape fare for a few hours. The invitations were for nine in the evening. Dinner started after a cocktail hour, and the party broke up between midnight and 1:00 a.m., or later when they had dancing after dinner.

Despite the pomp and the glamour, Barbara proved to be down to earth and easy to get to know. When I visited her at the Spanish embassy, Charles and Ginger enjoyed playing with the family pets in the backyard.

Somehow the term "backyard" didn't suit the spacious manicured grounds of a palatial embassy, and the word "pets" didn't quite suit the toddler chimp and infant gorilla. The ambassador inherited them from a prior resident, and he and Barbara had yet to locate an appropriate home for them.

One experience there wouldn't soon be forgotten.

"Just dress to play," she'd said. And we were to plan to stay for lunch. Her husband wouldn't come home before evening, and we could just have sandwiches out on the veranda.

It sounded delightful.

As usual, the gorilla playfully knocked Ginger over and gave Charles some good shoves. In the middle of an energetic romp, and after the gorilla and the chimp had muddied all four of us, a call came in from the ambassador's secretary.

"*Señora! Es urgente!*" An unexpected official visitor had arrived from Spain. The ambassador would bring him home in fifteen minutes. No problem. The embassy chef would whip up a gourmet lunch on the spot.

"Oooh. We'll hurry, Barbara. Go ahead and do what you have to do. I'll just get the worst of the mud off our clothes and we'll get out of—"

"Ab-so-lute-ly not! My personal guests are not going to be chased away. Don't even think about it. You're not leaving—and that's final!"

We cleaned up as best we could, while Barbara ran inside to change. She reappeared, calm, refined and ready for any guest.

We were seated, and luncheon was served. We must have made an amusing picture—the proper, not to mention serious, Ambassador Garcia Miranda on one side of the enormous banquet table flanked by his VIP guest and Barbara. Directly across from them, yours truly, between two muddied little people.

As we waited for the first course, Charles, who had quite a developed design sense for a five-year-old, asked, "What is this design on the plates? It looks Spanish."

Barbara said, "Indeed it is. This is a Spanish house and the design is the Great Seal of Spain."

Charles announced, "The Great Seal of the United States is much better because the eagle has leaves in its claws."

Barbara responded with a soft chuckle. I didn't look up to see whether the ambassador or his guest cracked a smile.

But this time Barbara was lunching at our house. As I checked in the freezer for our hot dog supply, I remembered I needed to get out my oil paints and brushes. Barbara and I both liked to work in charcoal, and we also wanted to try oil painting. I had a couple of books on working in oils and had a few still usable tubes of paint left from a previous abandoned effort. After lunch we would make a start.

Barbara asked whether I'd heard of a local artist named Gaspar Gomán.

I hadn't. She said he was well regarded, and "Wouldn't it be great if we could take some lessons from him, or at the least visit his studio?"

I said I'd love that but didn't think he'd be allowed to even see us.

"I've asked my husband to talk to President Macias and try to get special permission. No luck so far, but he said he would try again."

The prospects weren't good. Who in the world would Macias rather say no to than his country's former colonial power?

"Another hot dog, Barbara?"

# 21

## CHILD'S PLAY

*Ginger, still two* years old, typically played with her dolls and dishes, looked at books or rode her rocking horse. There were no children near her age, but Ginger seemed to enjoy her solitary play. And the absence of age-mates enhanced her speech development since her conversations were with older children and adults.

Her brother had a bit more adventure. We lived in a neighborhood of Nigerians, and Charles played with the neighbors' children, all a few years older than he. The parents stayed away from us, and we respected their boundaries. Even though they were Nigerian Igbos, and therefore not forbidden to have contact with us as the local citizens were, everyone feared talking to people affiliated with an embassy. You never knew when Macias would get a new idea in his head.

Although the adults were afraid to interact with Carl and me, they welcomed Charles into their homes. Many of their houses, in our same block, had walls and roofs of a patchwork of corrugated metal and sometimes sheets of cardboard. And Charles described dirt floors and no toilets.

Few days passed without a group of five or six boys and girls playing in our house or yard. They were accustomed to playing with what I regard as the best toys in the world—mud, sticks, rocks, water, string. They enjoyed Charles's Tonka truck to haul the mud, sticks and whatever else.

They made wonderful designs with our set of Cuisenaire Rods, the wooden rods in differing lengths and colors that were a hot new thing in math education. Math had been a mystery and a misery to Carl and me, and I had determined to help our children get a better start. Unfortunately, I hadn't purchased the teacher instruction book on how to use the rods. I finally gave up and they became just another toy.

If Carl and I were both away for a few hours, we often came home to find Charles had given away an entire case of colas or snack food we kept on hand for entertaining our tiny social circle. (He took after his dad.) Samuel never had the heart to stop him.

I enjoyed doing arts and crafts with our children, and reading and singing with them.

Any athletic play would be only with other kids. In my gym class in school, when teams chose sides, I was always the last person left and was met by loud groans from the team forced to accept me. And even though Carl had met tough qualifications to be on an air-evacuation team and to go through the rigors of high-altitude training, his only athletic activity in school had been distance running. He wasn't the roughhousing or playful type. As we were growing up, neither of our families had played anything more strenuous than croquet, darts or Ping-Pong. (Of course, a person could work up a good sweat at the Ping-Pong table.)

Besides taking Charles with him to work on occasion, Carl's way of engaging with the kids was sitting them down to have a serious talk—to explain things that were of vital importance to him. (Ginger's memory of the ritual goes back before her third birthday.) Was this the way his introverted personality allowed him to connect?

In the seeming safety of our neighborhood, Charles played in front of and near our house with his friends. But it was years before I knew about one of his adventures. On the corner near the house was a kiosk where he often bought Chicklets gum or some little treasure. This time he had saved his allowance and bought a pack of cigarettes. He slipped back behind the house, climbed up on our block wall, and tried one. He remembers it tasted disgusting to him and that he threw the rest away.

Charles had adventures away from home and neighborhood too. When Carl wasn't working on the mainland, he liked to include him in what he was doing, from simple things like driving Samuel home to grand adventures for a little boy. When a French warship made a courtesy call at the port, Carl took our son on board with him. Even today Charles remembers the formality, and the guns, which seemed enormous. He remembers the captain talking to him and giving him a bottle of Coca-Cola out of a small refrigerator in his quarters. For weeks, he did his best to assemble a naval-looking uniform and created paper hats modeled after the captain's. In fact, he made an entire collection of elaborate paper hats from photos of head wear from all over the world.

He often went with Carl to the chancery, where he hand-shredded papers for his dad. The chargé taught him flag protocol, and Charles loved lowering the flag at sundown.

The Nigerian playmates were always smiling and laughing. But arrests and beatings and disappearances were happening in Nigerian families, just not as much as within Guinean families. The things these children knew and talked about!

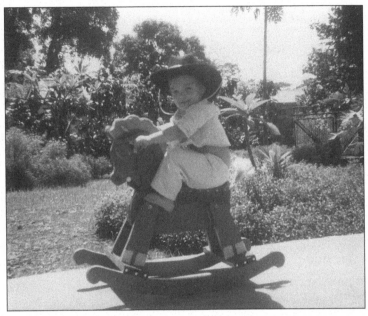

Ginger in our backyard in Equatorial Guinea, 1970

# *Reflection*

Through Five-Year-Old Eyes

every time he leaves
Dad says, "I'll be back soon"
I hear *soon*
soon

soon is a few minutes
a few hours
at most, a day

Dad doesn't come back
in a few hours
or a day
maybe days
can't trust "soon"
what if he's killed

now he's away again
didn't come back soon
what if he's killed

# 22

# THE OUTSIDE WORLD

*Feeling the isolation* a bit more than usual, I wrote a long letter on
August 28, 1970. This was one of those reserved for family members, but not to include Carl's parents.

> Sometimes it's hard to remember there's life beyond
> this dark movie we're living. But I'll try to give you a pic-
> ture of the few connections to the outside world.
> By phone: We do have a phone, but no real connec-
> tion to the outside. When Carl is working on the main-
> land (which is most of the time) we can't connect by phone
> even though he's in the same country.
> By mail: As you know, we use the diplomatic pouch,
> not the local post office, because:
>
> 1. (just a trivial matter really) You're not allowed to
>    put your own stamps on your letters. Reason: Who
>    knows?
> 2. Anyone buying a stamp is suspect. Reason obvious:
>    Buying a stamp indicates intent to mail a letter, which
>    indicates intent to plot against the government.

3. You must leave your letters at the post office, envelopes open. Reason: We have to be thoughtful and make it easier on the government. They read all mail to ferret out those "plots," and it's extra bother to have to untape the envelopes.

Three weeks ago, the government arrested and beat a Spaniard based on his letter that criticized the government of Equatorial Guinea (GOEG). They accused the man of plotting against GOEG, and he's being held for "public trial." That will be a kangaroo court for sure.

The director of television operations, also a Spaniard, was ordered to film a documentary presenting the evidence of this man conspiring to overthrow the government. He refused. They arrested him, beat him and expelled him from the country. Since Spain maintains the TV service here, the Spanish ambassador told Macias—if he goes, it all goes—finish! The government sent a special plane to Douala, Cameroon, to bring back the television director and his wife. Frankly, I can—not—imagine whatever possessed them to return!

Oh—and don't try to send us any periodicals. Those are forbidden. The embassy subscribes to a few US periodicals, which take about three weeks to reach us in the pouch.

By sea: I know I've already told you that because so many people fled the country, Macias had all the fishing boats destroyed, burned I hear, so no local can leave the island without his permission.

A Spanish ship, the *Ciudad Toledo*, comes to Santa Isabel once a month and then goes over to Bata in Rio Muni, Equatorial Guinea's bit of mainland. Carl and his teams sometimes take this, but it's not easy. The president signs, personally, for all travel by government employees.

A decrepit old Nigerian ship, the *King JaJa*, has begun picking up Nigerians desperate to go back home and makes the short run across to Port Harcourt or Lagos.

The local harbor pilot doesn't always pilot the ships. When he can't be found, the ships come into the harbor as best they can. Maybe with so little sea traffic now, that's not a big issue.

By air: The one big jet into and out of this place, Iberia's once weekly roundtrip Madrid–Santa Isabel creates the favorite social-sporting event. All the expats converge on the airport and the first half of the game begins. We watch people deplane and bet on how long this one or that one will stay. (Realistically, we have to wonder what fate will befall them while they're here.) The second half of the game two hours later is watching people depart and betting on whether they'll ever dare to return. Occasionally someone with one or another oil company comes in. They're taking readings or measurements of some kind. They seem to think there might be oil here. In fact, they must be pretty sure of it because someone said they're paying big bribes for offshore drilling leases. They never stay very long.

And now, the saga of Lineas Aereas Guinea Ecuatorial (LAGE).

LAGE's two little planes are scheduled for five round trips a week to Bata and two a week to Douala on the coast of Cameroon, if the pilot can wake the guy in the tower and get permission to take off.

We can no longer call the airport and ask whether a

flight has arrived or what time a flight will leave, because this is "strategic information." Once on board, nothing else is strategic, I guess, because a posted sign invites us to "visit the cockpit." Young women often accept that invitation and hang out with the Spanish pilots during the short flight.

A couple of weeks ago, Carl had to go to Cameroon on business, so we decided our family would go along and have a break from this place. One of LAGE's two planes had been in Madrid for repairs for a few weeks. The other had encountered preflight or in-flight problems on every single flight for the previous week, causing cancelations of half of them. Now the plane had been on the ground for maintenance for two days. LAGE said it was ready to fly again. Desperate for even a tiny taste of freedom, we boarded. We were roaring down the runway (well—I guess a Convair 440 doesn't exactly roar) for takeoff when the pilot cut back on the power and slowed to a stop. He revved the engines for a while and then headed back to the terminal. Everyone deplaned. Charles, Ginger and I would not have our little vacation after all.

But Carl had to go, as did Mike, a Second Secretary who has come for some reason on short-term assignment to our embassy. They felt they had no choice but to try again. After the maintenance crew worked on the engine for about an hour, Carl, Mike and a few other brave souls boarded again.

This time they were airborne but skimmed the top of the jungle as they headed out over the bay. One of the two engines backfired and then cut out. After turning and making it back to the airport, Carl and Mike chartered a plane to come from Douala to pick them up.

For their return on Tuesday, the only other day there is a link with the outside world, they again had to charter a plane. Carl and the embassy are requesting carte blanche for charter because they have to fly about once a week. These air experiences with LAGE are so frequent that Mike's famous definition of mixed emotions is, "leaving Equatorial Guinea—permanently—on LAGE."

But would you believe it? Week before last, when the Spaniard who is director of LAGE canceled a flight due to mechanical problems, the government claimed there was nothing wrong with the plane and arrested the man, beat him and gave him four hours to get out of the country.

Of course, The One True Miracle, as President Macias has dubbed himself, is too paranoid to fly on LAGE. Three weeks ago, to fly to the mainland portion of his own country, he asked Cameroon to provide a plane for him. When he visited Nigeria on Saturday before last, Nigeria Airways came and picked him up.

One more thing. I need to describe for you the scene when Macias made those two trips off the island this month. On the days of his departure, and his return: All stores and offices were closed; all government employees and all diplomats were required to be at the airport to bid him farewell and to welcome him back; all other Africans lined the road to wait for him; driving was prohibited anywhere in the town; walking from one part of town to the other was prohibited if it involved crossing the main road through town, where Macias would pass hours later.

At the home of one expat family who lives on that road, a policeman showed up before 8:00 a.m. He ordered them to close all doors and windows and keep them closed, from before the president left the palace for the airport until after he returned and was once again inside the palace, which turned out to be late in the evening.

Four of us who had gone to the Bahia for an early breakfast that day were trapped there for hours as well. (The president's office doesn't always give embassies advance notice.) The old hands here know to have a deck of cards at the ready at all times. I can now play gin rummy, hearts, and crazy eights. Not bad for a gal whose card-playing repertoire had been limited to Old Maid.

We'll have the same scene in town tomorrow because the president's going on another trip. In fact, this letter's departure will be delayed about nine hours because the chargé is due to carry the pouch out on the 8:00 a.m. flight. But—the president doesn't leave until 3:30 p.m., and <u>nothing goes before he goes.</u>

I love you—and miss you!

Bee

# 23

# BEATEN

*Several times a* week we got wind this person or that person was severely beaten. But "beaten" is such a generic word, isn't it? It didn't mean to me then what I came to learn it meant. There is much Carl never told me. The word can't in any way describe the reality. "Beaten" could mean beaten to within an inch of life, or at least until a person screams out a confession and implicates friends and family. It could mean beaten to death.

Often, no one knew what happened once a person was taken through the doors of the jails or prisons. Many were just never heard from again. Some were released with obvious brain damage. If someone who'd been arrested was later seen in the town with broken forearms and fingers, broken legs, burn marks, amputated limbs or a vacant stare, everyone knew not to ask questions.

# 24

# BUT WE WERE JUST OUT
# FOR A WALK!

*Besides Al and* Carman, Wolfgang Schorcht with the United Nations Development Programme (UNDP), his wife, Ulrica, and their two delightful daughters were our best friends in Santa Isabel, and we shared many happy hours and many a laugh. They were Argentinian, but of German descent and Germanic appearance. It was thanks to Wolfgang, the power plant advisor, that we had electricity when we did.

After the Spaniards were evacuated, to prevent total collapse of the infrastructure, Macias had invited the UN to send in technicians and advisors to shore up public services. Because some fluency in Spanish was required, most UN personnel were from Latin America. Unfortunately, El Presidente then prohibited their talking to the local people they had come to advise and train, so many UN experts gave up and left after weeks of futile waiting incommunicado.

One Sunday morning, Wolfgang and his family showed up at our door, their eyes not as bright as usual. Ulrica appeared shaken. Wolfgang was fed up. His report to his superior, the officer in charge of the UNDP in Equatorial Guinea, tells the story.

## Incident Report

On Saturday, August 15, 1970 at 9:23pm I went with my wife and two daughters, ages 10 and 12 years, for a walk. Our ten-year-old daughter had a dog on a leash. Approximately 75 feet from our house a uniformed policeman appeared and started kicking the dog, pushing my daughter around and hit my wife twice. He hollered something about "Mi Republica." We pretended not to understand Spanish. We then went to the police station and reported the occurrence.

As this is not the first time we have been harassed by local authorities (but had nothing done about it), kindly note that if there should happen any further unprovoked incident, I will feel myself relieved of my duties and depart from this country.

Carl forwarded a copy of the report to his own boss in Atlanta to show the environment in which we lived. His copy where he usually noted such things bears no indication of a response from CDC.

The Schorcht family and ours just got together more often. We shared more funny stories, and we laughed more. Most of the time.

# 25

# A SPY BEHIND THE TREE

*As much as* I missed my sister, I didn't want her to come for a visit. My notes reveal the situation:

> When people arrive here, unless they're on official or diplomatic passports, they're taken into a side room for a thorough search of luggage and person, under rifle. Then, throughout their stay, plainclothesmen follow them and record all their movements and the names of their contacts. After the traveler departs, their contacts then are picked up for questioning and are often beaten.
>
> Not every act is punishment. There are rewards too. Macias gave all the Guineans a day off when his wife was sick and he went to visit her in Cameroon. Once, he gave them a five-day holiday "because they had worked so hard." (Actually, the Nigerians are the ones who do all the work, but they get no days off. They're treated like slaves.)
>
> And then there was the art show with its ten entries. The second prize entry was a painting of a tiger waving a banner of PUN (the one political party). First prize went to a painting of President Macias looking down on Equatorial Guinea, rays of light streaming from his face.

Macias stations his personal watchdogs with their notepads outside our embassy chancery, the embassy residence and the homes and offices of all diplomatic personnel. They report who comes and who goes and when.

These men try to disappear behind a post or a tree, feigning one casual posture and another. Apparently, we aren't supposed to notice them. They seem at least sober, unlike most of the Guardia. There might be a remote chance of our being fooled—except for the attire. When not at work, even ambassadors in EG wear the cool cotton guayabera shirt, perfect for the steam bath we live in. But some of our watchdogs are off the pages of a fashion catalog. Black three-piece suits. Sometimes pinstriped. Buttoned vest. Crisp-collared shirt. Tightly knotted necktie. At three degrees north of the equator.

The watchdog assigned to monitor Carl's every move sticks to him like glue. He doesn't wear the three-piece suit since he's out in the jungle. He's supposedly a vaccination team leader. Even when Carl takes the once-a-month Spanish ship from the island over to Bata, Watchdog sees him off on Fernando Po and is on the beach on the mainland to await his arrival. How does Watchdog get there ahead of Carl? When Macias destroyed all the boats, he must have left one for clandestine trips.

Carl and the vaccination team always stay in the tiny hotel in Bata (six rooms, I think Carl said), and Watchdog always arranges for the room next to Carl. Last week, Carl changed rooms late at night, moving across the hall because the lock on his door was broken. Watchdog immediately traded rooms with Ricardo, Carl's administrative assistant, in order to move across the hall too. So subtle!

Experiences like this wound up recorded almost in code. I definitely would not write this in a letter that Carl's parents might see. Every time they heard of some unrest anywhere on the entire African continent, they called their congressman to insist on confirmation that we were safe. I suspect congressional staffers began to recognize their voices.

# 26

## BLACK BEACH PRISON

*Black Beach Prison* explains the empty streets. It explains the silence, the dull expressions. It explains a woman crossing to the other side of the street to avoid me, hoping no one would accuse her of interacting with a foreigner. It explains men following orders to stand for hours outside offices and homes. Macias and Black Beach, a monstrous place that swallowed the living, spawned the climate in which Carl worked and in which we lived.

As the crow flies, Black Beach Prison, one of the most infamous in Africa, stood a half mile from our house. But I never saw it. I did not know its exact location, did not know the extent of its cruelty. The screams were contained within its core. Only when going through Carl's files after his death, as well as consulting outside information, would I discover it was hidden an easy walk from where I lived—and discover the extent of what went on there.

Anyone, no matter how loyal to Macias, ran the risk of incurring his wrath. Every one of the few Equatorial Guineans we saw on the street—man, woman or child—every man who worked for us, risked the jaws of Black Beach.

The first step: arrest. Grabbed off the street or out of your home. No explanation. Just grabbed and thrown into Black Beach, or *Blabich* in pidgin. Next step: straight to incarceration, torture or execution. No interim steps such as booking, filing of charges or the niceties of a trial. No specified term of imprisonment stated. No right to a defense. Men or women could be imprisoned and executed merely because they were a relative of someone else who was arrested, with neither party given a reason. A family might never be told where the prisoner was held or whether he or she was still alive.

To prevent a family from providing food or moral support and to prevent contact with their own ethnic group, the Guardia often took those arrested on Fernando Po to the Bata jail over on the mainland, and vice versa. The Bata jail was nicknamed the "University" because so many college-educated citizens were imprisoned there.

Imprisonment in Black Beach meant being stuffed into a tight space, naked, often in total darkness and without room enough to lie down. It meant eating, sleeping and defecating in place. Having no way to clean oneself meant infections and rapid spread of disease. In a few individual closet-like cells, a prisoner had room only to stand. Guards kept constant watch and beat the prisoner any time he weakened and leaned against a wall.

Wrist and ankle fetters were tightened so they cut through to the bone and then bound together behind the body in tortuous positions the human body was never meant to assume. Once they had the prisoner in a position that would increase the pain of beatings, the jailers went to work. Guards and even fellow prisoners zealously wielded their instruments of choice—clubs, iron bars or machetes. Denied medical treatment after the beatings, many prisoners died of gangrene.

Naked, bound and blindfolded for days or weeks on end, without use of their hands or feet, prisoners were often forced to lap the meager ration of rice or bread up off the fouled, insect-ridden and rat-infested floor. Some sources report other gruesome details which have sickened me to read and which I could not bring myself to write down.

The International Commission of Jurists says prisoners were assigned to three groups based on seriousness of offense:

- *Brigade A*—political opponents—were labeled the most dangerous prisoners and received the most gruesome tortures. They were also put on heavy roadwork details, beaten while working and given no food or water. As they worked, they had to survive off fruit they could find in the forest.

- *Brigade B*—those who criticized the president or who had run-ins with the Juventud. Besides beatings, these prisoners were given punishing work details and no food, and they were at risk of being transferred to Brigade A.

- *Brigade C*—the common criminals—were better off than the rest. And they were "allowed" to help beat those in Brigades A and B.

Crammed with far more prisoners than it was built for, Black Beach's crowding intensified the torture. But when even the governor of Black Beach Prison considered it too crowded, he or Macias had simple solutions—further cut the daily ration of one cup of rice so prisoners starved sooner, or just execute another group of prisoners.

Execution did not provide an easy exit. I choose not to describe the methods, but they are revealed in gruesome detail in histories of Black Beach prisoners who lived to tell about it. Sometimes an official delivered an obviously brutalized body to a family, with a certificate attesting to death by natural causes. Or authorities broadcast on the radio a certain prisoner had committed suicide and that for security reasons the suicide note would not be made public.

In the grip of hideous tortures, it is not surprising many prisoners screamed out a confession and implicated innocent family and associates. But that seldom resulted in any relief of their own suffering or in their lives being spared. And Macias and his henchmen made sure the population heard what could face them if they happened to displease.

And so it happened this prison a half mile from our house got busier and busier. The streets I walked grew quieter and quieter.

# 27

# ISOLATION

*Macias's fiats were* unpredictable. After some new perceived threat, he amputated an entire limb of our miniscule body of about twenty-five possible associates. We already were forbidden contact with the local people. Now he decreed diplomats and other embassy personnel could not have contact with anyone connected to the United Nations. He claimed that UN advisors knew too much and might share it with diplomats.

We now could associate only with embassy types or the occasional expat visitor to the island. The hours of laughter and moral support with Wolfgang and the others were over. We'd have been reported by the telephone operator if we'd even tried to visit by phone. It was another life event that made it hard for me to remember the smallpox virus was our targeted enemy.

Carl and I were heartbroken to be deprived of a developing friendship with a UN couple from Colombia whom we had recently met. On their first visit to our home, the husband spotted the guitar Carl had given me and asked if he could play it. Of course I agreed, and he did a credible performance of a simple but lovely tune. After he finished, misty-eyed, he told us he had never before held a guitar. In long hours in Equatorial Guinea, he had run across a beginner guitar book and set out to teach himself to play. He drew a diagram of the frets and strings, life-sized on paper, and had practiced many hours on his paper guitar. Not a single eye was dry in our living room that night.

Now we and our UN friends could not even speak when we saw each other on the street. When we passed Wolfgang or Ulrica or our Colombian friends, our sad eyes spoke volumes, reaching for each other where our arms and voices could not.

In a few months' time, foreigners would be forbidden to travel outside the city limits of Santa Isabel. No driving down to the beach or the thirty miles down to San Carlos Bay or up into the cooler air of the foothills without express permission from the president. In effect, this would mean no one left the town because asking permission would invite suspicion of subversive intent. The isolation would be complete.

Carl was on the frontline of battle with microbes. Our family was on a frontline of a different sort.

# 28

# PRESSURE VALVE

*A part of* Carl's pay was a rest and recuperation leave (R and R) for physical and mental health. For official or diplomatic personnel assigned to difficult posts around the world, it helped the employee and family face the next year and remain productive. Two of the most debilitating hardship factors in Equatorial Guinea were the oppressive sense of isolation and the hostility of the host government.

Paris was the established R and R point for West African assignments. Before moving to Africa, we had planned to request permission to go to Kenya for R and R. But we discovered Kenya wasn't that much closer than Paris. You can fit the US three times in the band across the middle of Africa, below the Sahara and above southern Africa. Besides, travel within the African continent costs more than travel to and around Europe. Sometimes you "couldn't get there from here" and had to fly to Paris or Madrid to get to Nairobi. We chose to fly to Paris, do a road trip through Europe and fly from Madrid back to Santa Isabel. We needed a drastic change of scene.

When the day finally arrived, we were blessed that our twenty-minute flight from Santa Isabel to the mainland was without incident. Our flight from Douala, Cameroon, landed us in Paris after dark. By the time we arranged for a pension and ground transportation and actually got into a room, there was just time for a bowl of soup before falling into bed. Mentally, I hadn't yet left the jungle.

The next morning, we fished changes of clothes out of the luggage, got dressed and stumbled downstairs to the breakfast room for croissants with butter and jam. Now we could begin our R and R. We emerged into cool October air and—what was this? People. Smiles. Voices. People on the streets free to talk to each other. Charles and Ginger tugged us toward the bright colors and music of an ice cream cart and its huge bunch of balloons. Carl laughed. I laughed. And I laughed. I kept laughing, not happy laughing, crazy laughing—release of a safety valve on a pressure cooker. I clamped one hand over my mouth and one over my belly. Carl put his arms around me and squeezed tight to try to calm me, and I finally grew quiet.

I stole embarrassed glances in all directions, but no one was staring.

I was finally free. Free to dive into these surroundings.

We walked and walked and walked. For two days we walked everywhere to take in the major sights of Paris. Then we rented a car and headed for the countryside and a European road trip.

That little Renault could have been a Rolls Royce, so liberating were our drives free of the unpredictable whims of a dictator. Walk-up pensions with a shared bathroom down the hall could have been Buckingham Palace, so freeing was it to come and go with no one watching to record and report.

Aromas from village bakers lured us. We stopped beside the road and spread out our meals of bread and cheese and olives. We visited important sites everywhere we went. Carl's invariable detailed history lecture before we could leave the room each day would eventually be met with my impatient sighs and Charles's groans. Can we just go see it now? But what a privilege.

Not everything was sunshine and butterflies. The sudden change from the equatorial climate to Europe's chilly late fall weather, and perhaps exposure to different microbes, took their toll on the kids. We had to visit doctors in three countries during our road trip but were thankful we were *allowed* to see a doctor. A few days before our flight from Madrid back to Santa Isabel, Charles had to stay overnight at the Torreon US Air Force Hospital with a severe asthma attack. And they prohibited a parental overnight stay. Back then you didn't argue with hospital rules or military nurses.

Despite illness, the leave had provided a critical respite. Now, waiting in the Madrid airport at the end of October, I knew that in fewer than ten hours we would be back on the island. I started the process of steeling myself and marshaling what spiritual resources I could still muster. We knew the tension of living life on a wire with a capricious president unpredictably jerking that wire. We didn't know the other things we had yet to face.

—➤

Back in Santa Isabel, I made some notes about happenings since we left on R and R:

Carl is pleased with the program updates from Ricardo.

This evening we were over at the residence with Al and Carman to catch up on the latest. There's more of the same—chilling mayhem from Macias and his enforcers. A few more people PNG'd. Emily, the American WHO nurse who's been a good source of information for Carl over in Rio Muni, has had enough. Her efforts to conduct classes for healthcare auxiliaries have been frustrated by selection of students based on family or political ties, by absence of doctors available to contribute their expertise and by having no typewriter or other means to produce class materials. Emily is calling it quits a few months before the end of her nine-month contract. One more doctor on the mainland has high-tailed it out of here as well.

The North Koreans have brought in more people. Al still takes down their propaganda calendars. He gave us one.

So mayhem and commies are still the norm.

But. The most talked about event was what happened at the Spanish embassy. It seems a glamorous New York acquaintance of Barbara's came to the island for a few days, escort to a much older man, rather a Colonel Sanders type as I understand it—portly, white hair, mustache and goatee. Barbara held the usual big dinner party for all the expats. With everyone assembled, her houseguest made a grand entrance down the wide staircase—wearing a see-through film of a blouse, no bra, and two strategically placed little pockets. From what Carman describes, it sounds as if all the men were positively apoplectic and may never recover.

# 29

# MILESTONES

*Journal note: November 7, 1970*

When we got back to Santa Isabel last week, Nicolay Ivanov, Carl's work contact in the Soviet embassy, had sent us an invitation for a reception (it's tonight) celebrating the "53 *Anniversario de la Gran Revolucion de Octubre.*"

I picked out what I would wear! But all of a sudden, our State Department says we're not allowed to go. I'm so disappointed. That enormous Russian embassy, half a block up from ours, looks like a giant concrete bunker— cold and gray, with tiny windows. Al says they have at least thirty people in there. And they are bringing in more military advisors and a bunch of fishing trawlers (spy ships in disguise, no doubt), and may be building a naval base at San Carlos Bay. More residents of their embassy. They stay holed up inside that fortress. When they leave, it's never alone—always in pairs. I've been so curious.

But. It's not to be! Some hiccup happened (I don't even know what) in the tension between East and West, and our embassy has been instructed to boycott the reception.

The USSR will have to celebrate the "Glorious Revolu-
tion" without me.

*Journal note: November 9, 1970*

We celebrated Charles's sixth birthday today! I can
hardly believe it. I think he's happy to be back home and
with his friends after being so sick on R and R. Seven of his
Igbo friends enjoyed my pink elephant cake and had a great
time with the new toys we bought last month in Europe.
I recorded their singing. Besides "Happy Birthday," they
sang Christian hymns we hadn't heard in a long time. It's
too bad we don't have the freedom to meet with their families for church services.

Carl informed CDC that as of today's date, his program in Rio Muni has vaccinated 198,776 people against
smallpox. That's essentially the entire population of the
EG mainland.

Our embassy received word Charles de Gaulle died
today. The French ambassador will have a memorial mass
in the cathedral sometime in the next few days.

# 30

## MUSICAL MINISTERS—AGAIN

*When we had* boarded our Iberia flight to return from R and R, we didn't know just how soon we'd be back on the tightrope.

Following is an excerpt from a November 19, 1970, letter to William Foege, MD, director, Smallpox Eradication Program, CDC, Atlanta:

> From Carl Bloeser, Operations Officer, Equatorial Guinea:
>
> Once again we're having a week of "musical ministers," something we're all getting used to. The Minister of Health has been appointed Minister of Mines and Industries. The Minister of Mines and Industries is the new Minister of Justice, and of course that means that Dr. Rafael Obiang, the Minister of Justice and head of the Juventud, is the new Minister of Health.
>
> I think it would be fair to say that Dr. Obiang would win hands down any contest for Equatorial Guinea's most sinister man.
>
> He is out of the country now. I doubt I'll have the chance to see the new Minister before next week . . .

Certainly in the months to come, we will have to consider the political override to our programming in Equatorial Guinea. I will keep you informed of developments in the monthly activity reports.

# 31

# THE TERROR

*"Don't speak. Just* listen. Grab the kids and an overnight bag. Be ready in ten minutes."

Carl was calling from his office at the embassy. My husband could be a bottom-line person if he had to be, but this was different. His voice was wooden.

What was happening this time? Where were we going?

No opportunity to ask. Not safe to ask. The phone clattered back into its cradle as I ran to get our children and a few essentials.

Minutes later our family rode in silence through the sultry equatorial afternoon. The pungent smell of moist earth and decomposing undergrowth hung heavy in the air. As I hugged our two young children, my preoccupied stare settled on the American flag fluttering from the embassy car's flagstaff. It was not supposed to be flown unless the chargé or the ambassador was in the car.

No one spoke until we were safely inside the embassy residence and out of earshot of the driver, who we knew worked for the police.

Now my questions could be answered. We would spend at least this night under the protection of the flag. Dr. Obiang, the new minister of health, had let loose his gangs of armed youth against the Portuguese community, and they were slashing their way through the street three blocks away. Their clubs and machetes were demolishing shops and bludgeoning any Portuguese they could get their hands on.

Minutes earlier Carman had phoned the alert to the chancery. She had just left it herself and stumbled onto the attacks as she walked the few blocks to the residence. She escaped harm only because her hairdresser spotted her and rushed from the shop, screaming to the mob, *"No es Portuguesa! Es Americana!"*

We learned that farther up the West African coast, the citizens of Portuguese Guinea (later Guinea-Bissau) fighting for independence from Portugal believed they had sighted a submarine off their shores. Following just two days on the heels of a November 22 Portuguese-led attack on their neighbor, Guinea-Conakry, the sighting triggered a massacre there. Equatorial Guinea was making a show of solidarity.

Our embassy residence, with its spacious entry hall and curving staircase, stood on a slight rise a block from the harbor. Across the street sprawled the hacienda-style police station. The juxtaposition was jarring—serenity and hospitality on one side of the street, official torture and murder on the other. But on this night, most of the torment was a few blocks away.

Al telephoned President Macias and told him he had gathered all the Americans at the American residence, and we were under the protection of the United States government. He expressed confidence in Macias's ability to make sure no harm would come to us.

Nothing could ruffle either of the Williamses. They always appeared to be having a good time regardless of circumstances. A genuinely good time. Carman liked to "let her hair down"—I often pictured her in a hippie commune—but when she needed to observe protocol, she did it with flair. Even at the age of thir-ty-three, Al epitomized the calm and collected diplomat. His stance when in peril: "It's just part of representation."

Now he and Carl periodically cracked the door for an instant to look and listen for any up-to-the-minute sliver of intelligence. They otherwise talked, smoked Cuban cigars, drank the Spanish brandy Fundador and looked for things to laugh about.

The residence had moved from smaller quarters only a few weeks earlier, so I helped Carman hem new draperies for the mas-sive windows to the accompaniment of her sparkling laughter and conversation.

Charles and Ginger drew pictures, devised paper creations and enjoyed Sarah, the poodle. Years later Charles would report a memory of screams coming from the police station across the street. I didn't hear them, but perhaps his young ears were more sensitive than mine.

Sounds of furtive conversation and hollow laughter were coming from the far corner of the room. Al and Carl were discuss-ing the embassy's emergency and evacuation plan.

Seriously? This was our E and E plan? We would sneak down the arm of the bay to the Hotel Bahia and swim thirty yards to a tiny button of land that peered above the surface of the water. Did I hear correctly? Al lowered his voice, and I strained to hear the hushed exchange. I wondered at the few words I could make out.

I think I heard something about a rescue team and . . . a sub-marine? Would they really come for six little people?

Carl leaned forward, his balding head shiny with perspira-tion. He rubbed a hand across his chin, further muffling his voice, but I could tell he didn't like the plan. He knew I couldn't swim. And what about our kids? I did hear the words, "rather try rain forest..."

I was wishing we were a large enough embassy to rate US

Marine Security Guards. Or what about some kind of boat? I'd read somebody had invented an inflatable lifeboat. If only we had one of those.

So here we were, the six permanent Americans on this small island where tropical foliage and black sand beaches camouflaged the struggle for survival under a brutal and xenophobic government.

I felt oddly unafraid. I suppose because Al and Carman joked about the situation and took that diplomatic "just part of representation" attitude. But after they concluded we should all go to bed for what was left of the night, a stealthy disquiet settled beneath my take-anything-in-stride exterior. I was thankful for one thing: This was not, at least, one of the few times when Al had to be away and left Carl as acting de facto chargé d'affaires. I'd have hated for him to have to navigate this situation.

Sleep eluded me that night as the hands of the clock made their rounds. I picked my way through streets and alleyways of littered memories. I searched. I teased out threads. Why on earth had Carl agreed to come to this place after reading all those cables? And what did he see when he came and investigated in person?

I knew he couldn't share all that he learned. But whatever it was, he had said he was needed here. Being needed seemed to override everything else in Carl's mind. He welcomed tasks no one else would take on and thrived on accomplishing the impossible. It seemed to be something he could not resist.

He had grown up so differently from me. After his birth father left, his mother had to make the living. She placed Carl and his six-month-old brother, Kenny, in an orphanage for the five weekdays and took them home on weekends. At age two, Carl was the "big boy." He would get up in the middle of the night, slip into the crib room, and stand on tiptoe to look and make sure his baby brother was all right.

Two years later, their mother married a soldier from one of the rougher parts of New York City. He adopted the boys, and for the next fifteen years the family lived on a series of army posts. When Pop returned from Korea, a severely wounded survivor of the disastrous Battle of Unsan, his combat decorations couldn't hide the interior wounds that would never heal. Carl had never stopped being needed.

In one of the high-ceilinged guest bedrooms, his quiet, regular breathing told me he was sound asleep. I was wide awake.

I couldn't get comfortable. Tried not to wake Carl.

The brain I could not turn off ruminated in a continuous loop. I worried about our UN friends. Denied contact with embassy people, where could they find a safe haven tonight?

I wished I could hear my sister's voice. So far away, and no possibility of phone contact.

I didn't like what I'd heard of our possible escape options.

I turned my pillow over. The cooler surface soothed me. Maybe now I could sleep.

But no.

President Macias was on his way to slaughtering, imprisoning or driving into exile a third of his people. I had to put those dark visions out of my brain. I needed to pray. Why couldn't I pray?

I slipped out of bed and wandered in silence through the darkened expanse of the residence. Sometime in the wee hours of the morning, I crawled back into bed and fell into a fitful sleep.

Despite the night's vigil, neither escape option had to be employed, and in the morning, Al deemed it safe for us to return to our own house. We exited the embassy into a sunny day and surface calm. No sounds, as yet, came from the police station across the street. So far as I know, no one ever learned the body count for the night just passed.

Carl put the crisis behind him and pursued his objective with even greater resolve. At home, we continued with what passed for normal. I added more pieces to the jigsaw puzzle on our dining room table. Ginger drew pictures and played with her dolls. Charles played in his fortress, barricaded behind those cardboard blocks full of bayonet holes.

Two days later, Carl wrote in a follow-up to the November 19 letter to Dr. Foege that despite repeated requests to meet with the new minister of health, he had not yet succeeded. In understated bureaucratic-speak, chilling as I look at it now, he said:

> Dr. Obiang is just not available at present. He seems to be quite occupied at this time with Juventud activities. On Tuesday, November 24, the Juventud was unleashed on the Portuguese community of Fernando Po. It now appears that I may be able to meet with him on Monday, December 7 . . .
>
> I would suggest that authorized personnel review two classified cables concerning this matter at an early date: [Carl listed two classified cable identifiers.]

*The New York Times* referenced the events of our night in the embassy in an article printed six months later:

". . . one of Africa's most repressive governments . . . arbitrary arrests and beatings . . . legions of secret policemen, undisciplined soldiers and a militant youth squad maintain a climate of fear . . . One day someone might just disappear . . ." The writer said he was quoting a member of the "small diplomatic community that maintains nervous vigil here."

Regarding the attacks of November 24, he said,

> Currently they are whispering about what happened one
> day late last year . . . in a show of solidarity with Presi-
> dent Sékou Touré of Guinea . . . Bands of the Juventud, the
> government-sponsored youth movement, then poured
> through the streets of Santa Isabel, beating dozens of Por-
> tuguese shopkeepers and their families . . . although the
> government later deplored the pillaging, it was allowed
> to continue all day. . . . (*The New York Times*, "Equatorial
> Guinea Under Harsh Rule," by William Borders, May 10,
> 1971)

Later, a representative from the International Commission of
Jurists would report that the Juventud "was responsible for much
of the looting, killing, execution, torture, burning of villages and
informing on anyone." He says they practiced "violence as a line
of conduct generally aimed at terrorizing the population."

The new minister of health deserved his nickname, "The
Butcher."

## Reflection

weeping for what I know but can't hear
screams in the shanties, the rain forest, the prison

weeping for what I know but can't see
tortures by president, by militia
by guardian of health

Dr. Obiang, minister of health
a surgeon tortures with precision

# 32

# CAUTIONING CDC

*Carl wrote his* bosses at CDC about the fact that smallpox/measles program representatives from the Atlanta office had been in the area recently but had not visited his program in Equatorial Guinea. He needed their input. Why were they unwilling to come here and share the technical and consultative expertise Atlanta had to offer? Why did they always have Carl come out of the country and meet them somewhere else or ignore the Equatorial Guinea program altogether?

He also reminded Atlanta about censorship. Just as all mail taken to the post office had to be left unsealed, all incoming mail was opened and censored. Carl stressed that all mail should be sent by pouch.

And one last reminder to CDC. Any visitors to Equatorial Guinea should carry no documents related to the country:

> If a search is conducted, these documents could jeopardize our mission here. A recent example is the case of the dismissal of the president-director general of the prestigious French firm [Dragages] who entered the country with a briefing paper on EG. After review of the document, he was asked to leave the country.

# 33

# THE CULT

*Besides his long* history of paranoia and sadism, many believed Macias used the hallucinogenic iboga with increasing frequency. He was rumored to have encouraged the secretive Bwiti cult's re-emergence, with iboga known to play a major role in the cult's rituals.

Macias's rule grew more cruel and more bizarre. When one person was declared "guilty" (of no particular wrongdoing—just guilty), Macias often executed the person's husband or wife and might order their entire village burned. He murdered the husbands of women he took as mistresses. After ridding the country of a large percentage of the Bubi tribe and many Fang who displeased him, Macias turned his vicious attacks on his own clan and even his own family.

But Macias mesmerized the people with his rants. For one celebratory event, President Macias had invited Chargé d'Affaires Williams to attend. Al didn't know why Macias had singled him out, unless he hoped it would result in a report to the US State Department that Macias was adored by his people. Even though Al could not understand a speech delivered in Fang, he said it was clear that Macias's oratory held the huge audience "in his thrall."

Before many more months, they would be in his vise. Or in exile. Or dead.

# 34

# FINES AND WORSE

*Hastily scribbled snippets* in my files:

- Man fined 2000 pesetas for asking, "Is it true the president is away?"
- Hotel Bahía fined 15,000 pesetas (about $214 in 1970) w/ no prior notice because waiters still wearing pre-independence uniforms
- Man fined for bringing shoes into the country wrapped in a Spanish newspaper
- Spaniard arrested at airport and fined 4000 pesetas for wearing shorts
- Now no one allowed to drive or walk on the street or walkway that runs in front of presidential palace
- More Spaniards seen at airport on grass-cutting crew—cutting grass with scissors—as punishment and humiliation for some alleged offense
- More and more people are declared persona non grata (are PNG'd) and given a few hours to leave the country. (They're the lucky ones.)

- Frau Pleuger (tough independent German businesswoman) in town again—is in and out of Santa Isabel with her ship carrying her *apfel saft* (apple juice) she sells here—sometimes stays several months. Al says she's in and out of the presidential palace—no one seems to know why. On most recent trip—wonder if it'll be her last—passport and letter of safe conduct from the president confiscated—has been held several weeks against her will.

  (We would later read that a German businesswoman, Mrs. Pleuger, must be the very same woman, wife of Friedrich Pleuger, a West German diplomat in Ghana, brought in products to sell, and bought 2,732 tons of cacao. Macias reportedly accused her of treason following an argument over the quality of both her product and the cacao. He demanded four million pesetas, the equivalent of $57,600, for her release. There was a campaign in the international press on her behalf, but Macias raised his price, and the Pleugers finally gave him twelve Mercedes Benzes to gain Mrs. Pleuger's release with a deportation.)

- Over in Rio Muni (mostly impenetrable jungle with national boundaries difficult to detect), a few French soldiers wandered across border from Gabon—arrested by Guardia—French ambassador apologized for error—president said okay, mistakes happen. But Guardia picked up employee of French company Dragages—beat him severely. French ambassador protested. The president said France had violated Equatorial Guinea's territory, he wouldn't put up with this kind of thing and Equatorial Guinea would send forces to France.

- Last week man in a bar walked over to another man—asked for a light for his cigarette. The man he approached was minister of something-or-other, but he didn't know that. Minister of justice was also sitting there—jumped to his feet—said, "What do you mean asking a minister to light your cigarette? Have you no respect for your leaders?" Hit the man, handcuffed him, took him away.

# 35

# MAY I HEAR FROM YOU
# AT AN EARLY DATE?

*Carl started to* worry that our children and I might need to be evacuated. On December 18, 1970, he wrote Bob Hogan, CDC's chief of operations for our area, requesting information:

> Dear Bob:
> If you have routinely been receiving cable traffic out of Santa Isabel, you know that we're living and working in a deteriorating political environment. In the event my family should have to be evacuated, could you give me some idea as to what separate maintenance rules and regulations would apply, if any? If evacuation of my family is recommended by the embassy, I would probably move them on a temporary basis to the Canary Islands or to Spain.
> I am not anticipating evacuation at this time, but I would like to have this information available in the event

something should happen during the remaining months of my assignment in Equatorial Guinea.

May I hear from you at an early date?

Sincerely yours,

Carl H. Bloeser

Operations Officer

Equatorial Guinea

[Carl had a practice of writing the date of response in the upper right corner of his copy of any letter or memo. There is no such notation on this document and no response document in Carl's archives.]

# 36

# JESUS HE BEEN BORN

*I rather enjoyed* the quiet Christmas of 1970. Just simplicity and nothing tempting us to spend money. The kids hung stockings. We made little gifts for each other and for Al and Carman's family. Their children, Mark and Katharine, were home from boarding school in Dakar.

I helped Carman prepare a semi-traditional meal. Having their kids with us was a delight. They shared tales from the outside world, and we were eight Americans for Christmas dinner!

The most heartwarming thing that season came on a Christmas card—the nativity story in Nigerian Pidgin English. I love that pidgin languages around the world bring people together, enabling communication among people from different tribes— who have different native languages. And so I loved this reading of the oh-so-familiar biblical account. It felt fresh and vibrant.

*Jesus He Been Born for Bethlehem*

*For them time when Caesar Augustus he been put law for he people, say: make all man them go walka for them own father-town for write he name.*

*So Joseph and Maria . . . them been go walka for Bethlehem. But them no been look no place for sleep for inside the town. So them been sit down for some sheep-house. For the same night-time, Jesus, whe He be the Son of God, He been born for there. Maria he been put some bikin [baby]-cloth for Jesus . . . been put the Bikin Jesus for some chop box.*

*The Angel, he been talk for the sheep-boys how Jesus He done born. Onetime some Angel for the Lord, he been talk say: "Make you no fear. Me I de bring for you good news for glad plenty. For this same night-time so, some Helper He don born for you, He be Christ the Lord. Make this i go be sign for you: You go look some bikin-cloth, and whe de sleep for inside them box."*

*For same time how Angel, he been finish for talk, plenty angel them begin for praise God; them been sing say: "Glory be for God whe live for up, and glad for all people for ground, whe them de get good heart."*

# 37

# HIGH-LEVEL DIPLOMACY

*Excerpt from our* Christmas newsletter:

Before I close out our letter for another year, I have to share one of our favorite stories. Santa Isabel is like a microcosm of the world. When you have a one-square-mile capital city with nine embassies and diplomatic missions—and only one restaurant—world politics play out on a mighty small stage. The conversational buzz comprises quite a mix of languages. For watching and listening for global political currents, we have ringside seats.

In October, Equatorial Guinea, increasingly unfriendly to the West, extended diplomatic recognition to communist China, and four diplomats arrived from Peking. But as the United States recognizes the Chinese nationalist government in Taiwan and not "Red China," and tries to persuade the rest of the world to follow suit, our embassy has been instructed not to acknowledge them in any way. We see them almost daily, either at the Hotel Bahia or in one of the not-yet-boarded-up shops, but we don't look at them and they don't look at us. Except, of course, to notice where each goes and who each talks to—and report back.

For instance, we know when the Chinese and Russians are and are not speaking to each other.

The Chinese Communists (Chicoms for short) have been here nearly three months now. Last week our ambassador came over from Cameroon for his quarterly visit, and on the day of his departure, he took the entire American community—all six of us—to lunch at the Bahia. During our meal, the four Chinese arrived. They walked right past our table as usual, but we didn't look at them, and they didn't look at us. They settled in at the table nearest ours, also as usual, but we didn't look at them, and they didn't look at us. And lunch proceeded.

But—not as usual—Ginger, not quite three years old, finished eating and slipped down from her chair. She stepped to a post between our table and theirs and started peeking around it, first one side, then the other. I don't know—she must have felt a connection because she has an uncle who is Chinese. I wasn't sure what to do. I looked to Ambassador Hoffacker, and he signaled me to do nothing. We all pretended to ignore our toddler's flagrant breach of an official order from the US Department of State.

The four Chinese gentlemen resolutely glued their gaze on their bowls of food. But Ginger was not to be deterred. When they could take it no longer they started batting eyes, wiggling fingers, chuckling. Finally, the principal Chinese diplomat looked over and smiled and nodded to our ambassador. Our ambassador smiled and nodded in return.

Much love to everyone, and a Merry Christmas, from Bee, Carl, Charles and Ginger

The following April, 1971, diplomatic history was made when the US Ping-Pong team was invited to visit the People's Republic of China. *Time* magazine referred to the event as "the ping heard 'round the world." Americans began to read about Ping-Pong diplomacy. And then! President Nixon announced, to the astonishment of all and to the horror of many, that he would visit China. Well. In our house we say, "Ginger was before Ping-Pong."

# 38

# THE *KING JAJA*

*Their steps swift* and silent, a group of Nigerian Igbo slipped from the shadows behind our house into the next alleyway in the direction of the port. They were fortunate ones who had evaded detection as they made their way from the plantations, through the rain forest, and from the edge of the forest into the alleyways of tiny Santa Isabel. Now they huddled and listened for word of the decrepit Nigerian ship's next arrival.

In the early weeks of 1971, the *King JaJa* was shuttling back and forth, ferrying Nigerians out of Macias's murdering reach and back to their homeland. The numbers hiding out in the town waxed and waned based on the *JaJa*'s arrivals and departures. And as the numbers swelled, so did the tension and the potential for trouble.

Seventy thousand Nigerians, mostly Igbo, had made their living and their lives here on the cacao plantations under Spanish colonial rule and in the few years since, but thousands now found it intolerable to stay. The departure of the Spanish left many fincas abandoned, and this left Nigerians without work. The rain forest reabsorbed the land.

But who suffered more, the unemployed or those with jobs? Macias gave the fincas that were still operational to his friends.

Physical and mental abuse increased by the day. And after the Spaniards left, wages were first greatly reduced and then were paid only sporadically. Macias ordered the murder of at least ninety-five Nigerians who had the temerity to demand their back pay. It was neoslavery.

The end of the Nigeria-Biafra War also drew the Igbo back to their homeland. Their fellow Igbos were rebuilding Eastern Nigeria. Many on Fernando Po were eager to go home and join the effort, as uncertain as their future there might be.

Thankfully, Samuel seemed somehow protected from the conditions that plagued his countrymen who worked the plantations. He didn't try to hide. But when Carl wasn't over on the mainland, he took the truck and drove him home more often these days. How long would Samuel hold on before he tried to get out, especially once we left? People who could be potential employers of household staff were fleeing Fernando Po. The Soviets brought in their own people, and I guessed the Chinese and North Koreans did the same. I prayed that when the time came, Samuel would get away unharmed.

When the Igbo huddling around our house and in other alleys in town got wind the *King JaJa* had been spotted on the horizon, they mobbed the Nigerian embassy and then the docks. On the pier, drunk soldiers beat them and tried to grab their meager possessions. We heard that at least one Nigerian was bayoneted to death.

Fear-gripped crowds surged onto *JaJa's* decks. The ship built to carry three thousand sometimes sailed with twice that number. The Nigerians who didn't make it on board stayed on the alert for whispered news of the ship's next arrival.

But for Ricardo, and for the other Guineans, there was no avenue of escape.

# PART III

# THE TURNING POINT

# 1

## THE CALM BEFORE . . .

*It didn't seem* fair. My escaping the tension while the rest of my family stayed in Equatorial Guinea, but Carl was going to be in Santa Isabel for the week, and I needed to see a doctor for my physical. I had to admit it would be a relief to get away from the island. The kids would be in good hands. Samuel would keep the household running smoothly and be sure Carl had clean clothes. The necessary trip could be turned into a nice break for Mom.

So I packed a bag for four days—one-day travel time to Yaoundé, Cameroon, one day to see the doctor, one day to wait for the next plane back and one more day for the return trip.

After the twenty-two-minute flight to Douala, several hours' layover in Douala, and the final leg to the capital, I stepped into the cool mountain air of Yaoundé.

That's when I first met the Bradleys. They were pushing an empty wheelchair and had thought they might even need a stretcher. They hadn't been told why I was coming, a communication lapse that triggered the first of many laughs.

Dr. Martin Bradley was the smallpox/measles program's medical epidemiologist for Chad, Central African Republic, the Congo, Cameroon and Equatorial Guinea. Carl had met him at area meetings and liked him. Martin's wife, Dr. Joyce Bradley, provided care for American embassy personnel and their families. Most physicians don't house their patients, but these smallpox colleagues insisted I stay with them. (I would later learn the Bradleys would have done the same had I been any stranger in need of shelter.)

As we drove through town, I was jarred by car horns and bicycle bells, by the shouts of roadside hawkers and taxi drivers and the voices of just—being. I'd gotten so accustomed to silent streets I'd forgotten the sounds of life.

The next day, I accompanied Joyce on her visit to a mission hospital out in the bush. We drove down any road we wanted. We talked with whomever we wanted. We stopped at roadside stands to buy fruit, and vendors chatted with us. And all around us laughter. So much laughter. It was a tonic. I found my smile muscles still worked.

After that boost to my spirits, another came in the comforting presence of the US Marine Security Guards at the entrance to our embassy, Ambassador Hoffacker's resident post. In her upstairs clinic, Dr. Joyce pronounced me in good health, and now I'd have one more day in her mirth-filled home while I waited for the next return flight.

The morning of my departure the embassy gave me a diplomatic pouch to carry back to Santa Isabel. Before I walked out and climbed the steps to the little plane, I think I said something to Joyce about the laugh therapy equipping me to soldier on.

# 2

# INTERNATIONAL INCIDENT

*The familiar soup* of an equatorial afternoon surged up from the tarmac and pulled me into it as I came down the steps of the Convair 440. The date was February 4, 1971.

I resisted the Guinean official who tried to take the diplomatic pouch I was carrying, gratefully handed it over to Al Williams, and then looked beyond the Guardia, with their semiautomatic rifles. My husband stood rigid outside the shabby terminal. Carl's jaw set, his feigned smile tight, he shifted awkwardly. *He's trying too hard to look casual. Something's up.*

The customs shed's dim light obscured any clues I might have gathered from a closer look at his face. I claimed my bag and ran the gauntlet of government officials. When we got to the truck, Carl gave me a perfunctory peck on the cheek, his furrowed brow appearing carved in stone as he turned the key in the ignition. He showed minimal interest in asking about my trip, and I forgot the funny things I had planned to tell him. I could see from his face that asking questions would have to wait.

Lemongrass lined the island's one well-maintained road, and the citrus-like aroma floated in and penetrated the silence as we rode along the edge of the rain forest into town. When we reached Santa Isabel, the lemony scent yielded to odors from garbage accumulating in empty lots and from the mold of neglected or abandoned buildings. The streets were dead quiet, all the more noticeable after four days' absence.

When we arrived at the house, I noticed Samuel had misplaced his smile. After I hugged Charles and Ginger and gave them the little treats I had brought them, Carl asked Samuel to take them to the backyard to play.

"Bee, we need to talk."

We sat across from each other. Carl put his palms together in front of his chest and tapped the sides of his index fingers on his pursed lips. This gesture of his always meant something was coming I wouldn't want to hear. After what seemed like an age, he continued.

"It's time to get you and the kids out of here."

I stiffened and sat up on the edge of my chair. What had happened this time?

After another long silence, Carl began. He said he had been working in his office at the embassy, the children at home with Samuel, when it all started. So the first part of the story was related to Carl by Samuel.

Charles and a neighbor girl had been on the front porch, making little bows and arrows with small branches, twigs and rubber bands. Charles was on the sidewalk around the corner from our gate with an eight-inch bow and longer arrow when two Guardia came walking down the street. And he shot at them. One of the Guardia ordered Charles to come to him. Charles yelled, "No!" He ran to the porch, the Guardia followed him, Charles dashed into the house screaming, and Samuel bolted the door. Terrified, Charles hid under the dining table and barricaded himself with the legs of the chairs.

One of the Guardia pounded on the door. "I want that boy! Give me that boy!"

Samuel refused to unbolt the door. He told the man he would have to go to the American Embassy and talk to Carl. Our dear, loyal Samuel. Africans here were tortured or killed for much less serious insults to the government—and he knew that. Samuel had risked his life for us.

The two Guardia finally left, but one returned to our house a little later. He pounded on the door and demanded once again that Samuel hand Charles over. Samuel had phoned the embassy as soon as the man left the first time. Carl had rushed home, and now he asked what the problem was.

"That boy is making weapons dangerous to the Republic of Equatorial Guinea."

When Carl did not succeed in placating the Guardia, he called Al, who arrived within minutes. By this time playmates and about twenty curious adults had gathered outside the gate.

On our front porch, our chargé d'affaires defused the crisis. His opening gambit, good-natured palaver, was the setup for diplomatic thrust and parry. Al snapped the arrow into two pieces and brushed his hands together in a that-settles-that gesture. "There. That'll show that kid. He won't be doing that again." Al then turned and admonished Charles to "never again shoot a toothpick at a soldier."

Despite the accusation of Charles threatening national security, with the "weapon" now destroyed, he was not arrested. But fear on the part of his friends' parents kept the playmates away.

—➤

The story Carl told me sounded more like a bizarre movie than reality. My head had become semi-comfortable in the sand. A sense of detachment from my fiction-like life. And despite the ever-present stress, it seemed danger was strangely exhilarating.

Others have written of similar contradictory feelings in dangerous settings—something about the adrenaline.

But now the Guardia had tried to arrest our son. This was not a Hollywood story. This was a dangerous time in a dangerous place. Regretfully, we could do nothing about the atrocities committed by this regime against tens of thousands of innocent people. But we could do what was necessary to protect our family. It was time to go.

Carl wanted us out of Equatorial Guinea. I sent a plea by the next diplomatic pouch to Martin and Joyce Bradley. As physicians, could they help get us out?

The professional diplomat had put a light spin on the situation, but Charles doesn't believe he was playing around when he shot that arrow. In his memory he fully intended a justified attack against a brutal enemy.

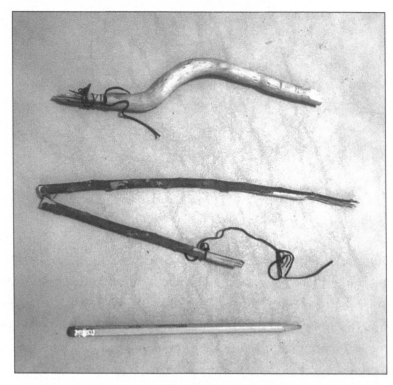

The Weapon

# 3

# TIME TO GO

*The year 1971* had dawned with increasing violence by Macias against his own people. His attacks on foreign nationals were more frequent and expanding to take in nationalities besides the Spanish and Portuguese. As February was getting up a head of steam, our own family had been assaulted. I typed a letter to my sister and made carbon copies for ourselves and Carl's brother. A few bits escaped the edges of the page as I crammed our lives and our apprehensions onto my one sheet of onion-skin paper.

February 9, 1971

Here's a small installment on the newsletter I've not finished! I'm trying to get all the news together, but everything is so up in the air all the time and I hate to send out a cliffhanger. This will be almost in telegraph form—I'll write more detail later.

We've been witnessing a communist takeover [since October.] The North Koreans have been bringing in more people (about nine in their embassy now). Communist Chinese has established an embassy and now have at least twelve people here. The Russians now have over thirty and the president has bought a Russian plane with two crews for his own use. The great favorites are the Chinese. They get really special treatment. The government even furnished them a car on which to fly their flag. They're active for sure—not wasting any time.

An average of four to five people a week are PNG'd. I think I wrote you that Mrs. Pleuger, the German businesswoman who came back in here with a letter of safe conduct from the president, had the letter and her passport confiscated and spent several weeks here against her will. This was on BBC and in the *New York Herald Tribune*. Last night the hotel was nationalized. The Nigerians have been crowding around the Nigerian embassy by the thousands, and yesterday they were nearly rioting. They're desperate to get out of EG, and many difficulties stand in their way. The honorary British vice consul who had lived here for seventeen years left, escaped, I should say, and was rather grateful to get out alive and unharmed. I've already told you about the riots against the Portuguese and our being sheltered in the embassy. Etc., etc., with several other things I can't write about. The tension is growing, and the only people that seem to feel at ease here are the Russians, North Koreans, Communist Chinese, and a man from Haiti.

Last week I was over in Cameroon for a few days, and the kids stayed here with Carl. They made out just fine, but there has been a little incident—long story—write you the details in the next few days. And I don't know whether this really happened, but Carl understood Al to say that when their son Mark (age 10) was home for Christmas, a policeman hit him and took his bicycle. Al and Carman are beginning to get nervous now too, and that's really saying something. A couple of nights ago, I heard Carman tell someone that she was glad their children weren't here—for their own safety. So then when Carl told them that he wants me and the kids out of here within thirty days, they said they didn't see how we could do anything else.

At this point we haven't made a definite decision as to where we will go. We want it to be Yaoundé, Cameroon, as our ambassador is there. I could be in touch all the time and wouldn't be sitting somewhere in the States waiting three weeks for news. However, the Cameroon is extremely expensive and we may have to go to Las Palmas in the Canary Islands. Carl's contract will be up at the end of September. . . . Have to close now, as they're about to close the pouch. I'll keep you informed. Recommended reading: Jan 31 *NY Times*—"China Finds an African Friend in Tiny Equatorial Guinea."

'til later,

Bee

Even if I was out of the habit of praying, I hoped—no, I knew—that my sister prayed for us. I still wanted those prayers.

# 4

# EXIT

*My February 7* letter to Drs. Martin and Joyce Bradley told them
about the attempt to arrest Charles and appealed for their help in
getting our children and me to Cameroon. I expressed an urgency, but I hadn't dreamed they would—or could—move so fast.
And I had no idea whether State would approve bringing us to
Yaoundé.

I knew of State Department evacuations of groups of families
from places like the Congo and a few individual evacuations. But it
appeared that to qualify, you had to have bullets flying over your
head, a serious illness that could not be treated at post, or a mental
breakdown. Well, whatever it took. Within a week Ambassador
Hoffacker ordered us evacuated to Cameroon. The kids and I flew
out of Santa Isabel on February 16, and Martin and Joyce met us at
the Yaoundé airport.

The day before we were evacuated, Charles, worldly-wise now
beyond his six years, hurried in the door with one last bit of intelligence whispered to him through the hedge by a neighborhood
playmate.

"Mom, my friend said the government's gonna kill every person in this country."

# PART IV

# THE LONG SHADOW

# 1

# GUNBOATS

*About the time* the children and I were landing in Yaoundé, Carl faced a tense situation back in Santa Isabel. Al and Carman had come out on our same flight for a business trip, and Al had once again designated Carl acting de facto chargé d'affaires. The only American in the country, Carl just hoped nothing would happen that couldn't wait for Al's return.

Tensions were ratcheting higher in Santa Isabel. The *King JaJa* waited at the dock and had been there for several days as Macias stalled on allowing the ship to take on the thousands of passengers jamming the port.

About three hours after our plane took off, two gunboats appeared on the horizon unannounced, making for the harbor, signals flashing. Their markings could not be seen. Speculation and some degree of panic spread among those watching from the Bahia or the cliff overlooking the harbor, and Carl says he mulled the familiar question, "What on earth am I doing here?"

As it turned out, Ghana was just making courtesy visits at various African ports. After much ado, one boat was permitted to dock, and the next night the captain hosted a state reception on board. Carl represented the United States.

That wasn't his only embassy duty before Al returned, because

an American traveling around Africa and curious to see Equatorial Guinea landed at the airport. Not surprisingly, the police confiscated his money and passport. Carl never ceased to amaze me.
He persuaded the government to return both and allow the man
to leave the country, which I thought was quite a feat for a CDC
man. If the traveler only knew how fortunate he was to leave with
his person, if not his curiosity, intact.

# 2

# THE DOCTORS BRADLEY

*A retreat for* a just-evacuated family. That's what this frazzled wife needed. Until the State Department untangled the red tape for a housing allowance for our children and me, Martin and Joyce Bradley opened their home. Their three-bedroom house now sheltered three adults and five children. The Bradley home was always open to wayfarers, of whom there were many, so the Bradley children were adept at accommodating outsiders in their lives.

Martin and Joyce were the most unimpressed-with-themselves physicians I had ever met. "Down-to-earth" doesn't even come close. They were both brilliant, dedicated physicians but had a lighthearted approach to life. Joyce was never at a loss for one-liners herself, but Martin, to the casual observer, had not a single serious bone in his body. He'd wear a Groucho Marx glasses-nose-mustache disguise. He'd play ruffles and flourishes on his kazoo prior to some slapstick feat—*ta-dah!* He'd act like a vampire to torment a waitress trying to take his order. Stupid stuff. We would laugh so hard our sides ached. And I had thought Carl's sense of humor was bizarre!

The truest way to describe Martin, for those old enough to remember, is to evoke the 1970's satirical book, movie and television series *M\*A\*S\*H*, about a mobile army surgical hospital. The writers had to have followed Martin around to write the iconic character of Hawkeye Pierce. In fact, Martin had served in a MASH unit in Vietnam, so maybe there was a hidden camera. Some years in the future, Colonel Martin Bradley, MD, would turn down a star because neither he nor his wife wanted Joyce Bradley, MD, to have to play the role of general's wife.

This home was therapeutic—the perfect place in which to decompress. Charles and Ginger had the Bradley children to play with. I learned new skills from Joyce. She had enormous creative energy for cooking, knitting, crafts, games (with her ten-month-old in a carrier on her back) and fun outings. Yaoundé had a lively feel, the grocery stores had wonderful French cheeses and the air was invigorating. The knots inside my body were beginning to unravel, one tangled nerve at a time.

# 3

# AFTERSHOCK

*First came the* sound of his wild flight up the stairs and then my son's frantic eyes as he ran into the guest bedroom, slammed the door and locked it. Breathless and quivering, he shoved the barely audible words into the space between us.

"Mom. The police. The police are here."

Panic. He'd been playing happily just a moment earlier.

I tried to reassure Charles, and he and I started down the stairs just as Ginger started up the stairs in as fast a run as a barely three-year-old can manage.

"Oh! Oh! The police are coming to get me!"

Charles, Ginger and the Bradley children had been playing in the front yard when a group of Africans arrived and entered the yard. The group was just there to see Joyce for routine vaccinations. But unfortunately for Charles, two of the men were wearing uniforms of some kind.

We had hoped to shield our children from fear of the police. I'd often read them a little story popular at the time, *Peter Pat and the Policeman*, about the kind officer helping Peter find his way home. But our feeble efforts were drowned out by overheard conversations and the undertow of our own stress, not to mention direct interaction with the Guardia. And what about the stories heard from local playmates—stories of an uncle or cousin or friend who had been tortured or who had vanished?

My heart wanted to stop as I registered my first true insight into Charles's trauma at the hands of the Guardia. I had agreed it was time to get out, but my hearing of the attempted arrest was secondhand. Charles had gone back to his typical play, and Ginger hadn't seemed upset. The event had become part of the fictional feel of life in Equatorial Guinea. The tale had even taken on a co-medic absurdity with frequent retelling.

Now I was holding two trembling little children. I couldn't hug them tightly enough. I'm their mom. I was supposed to pro-tect them. If I hadn't been relaxing here in Cameroon, could I have done something?

The worst of it was not knowing how long their fearfulness would last. If only I could rewind, delete memories. If only . . .

---

At an embassy reception in Yaoundé, a State Department vis-itor out from Washington was introduced to me. "Oh, you're the mother of the little boy who nearly created an international inci-dent!" He told me Chargé d'Affaires Al Williams had detailed the incident and his destruction of the dangerous weapon in a cable. "It's framed and hanging on the wall of the cable room at State," he said.

I've never seen the cable, but I still have the broken weapon.

# 4

# SETTLING

*It's one of* the blessings of life that periods of intense trauma are replaced by the everydayness of life. Charles and Ginger could play with children near their own age, and Charles attended the international kindergarten, his first opportunity for school since we left Kano. We continued to have new diversions in and around Yaoundé, and the Bradleys were nothing if not entertaining.

One afternoon at the Bradley home, Joyce and I stepped into the front yard, where the kids were playing. I pointed up the dusty road to what looked like a huge oil spill. It reached from one side of the road to the other. But then, as we watched, the thing was oozing toward us.

"Oh, for—! *Army ants!*" Joyce raced to a storage room to grab the kerosene.

This one colony of aggressive foragers could contain as many as twenty million ants. Its march was relentless—steadily closing the distance between them and our yard.

We had to keep the ants from turning into the driveway and getting to the house. At newcomers' orientation, expats were told the best defense against an army ant disaster in the house was to use kerosene to divert the raid in the first place. If they got into the house, we could only grab children and pets and get out, because if we disrupted their formation they'd scatter, be unable to reorganize, and become permanent tenants.

Army ants consume snakes and other small animals as well as prey closer to their own size. If you leave them alone, the army will stay organized, go on through the house and be on their way. And—big bonus here—your house will be clean as a whistle. Army ants, also called driver ants, and their marches and bivouacs are a fascinating topic. But we preferred not to have our own personal experience with the subject.

In seconds, Joyce was back with the kerosene and poured a wide strip between the two concrete pillars at the driveway entrance. The horde would soon reach the corner of the Bradleys' yard. We stood frozen and fascinated as we watched the army's leading edge begin its incursion toward the gate. I picked up Ginger and took Charles's hand. Joyce had her youngest in his carrier on her back and her other two by the hand in case the ants penetrated our defenses.

The army marched to the kerosene barrier and continued along its edge. The lead troops curved back toward the center of the road and the army marched on toward its next raid. By dusk it would need to bivouac, 120 million tiny legs, linked together, looking like a black hammock in the trees. We would leave it to others to follow them with notepads and cameras to document this bit of animal behavior.

Our stay at the Bradleys' stretched into six weeks, by which time we were all ready to have our own space. But a bond had formed that became a lifelong friendship.

What a blessing that State finally approved an apartment for the kids and me. Its living–kitchen area and one bedroom were tiny but comfortable. The wall separating us from the neighbors ended about eighteen inches from the ceiling. On the other side was a young Lebanese couple, so I enjoyed the aromas of anise, lemon, garlic and olive oil. With typical Lebanese hospitality, they invited us for dinner, and I soon added tabbouleh, hummus and couscous to my list of favorites.

I think back with compassion for the couple on the other side of that partial wall. I've always loved to sing. My bedtime songs for my children were never Brahms, but "Tumbling Tumbleweeds" and "Summertime," with another blues tune or two thrown in. (I'd taken lessons from an African American voice coach one semester and developed a love of the blues.) During the day I filled the air with the three-chord songs of my entire guitar repertoire—"If I Had a Hammer" and "Where Have All the Flowers Gone."

Charles had no opportunity to fold the embassy flag in the evenings as he had enjoyed in Santa Isabel, but he got to know the US Marine security guards at the embassy in Yaoundé and quickly took to them, uniforms and all. For some reason, he seemed to sense they were there to protect us. Perhaps the fact they were in our embassy, with the familiar great seal and the flag, said to him, "You're safe here." I could only guess.

Charles built ships from scrap lumber and explained each step in his process to classmates at morning kindergarten. While he was at school, Ginger and I went to the embassy to check for messages from Carl and news of Santa Isabel. We either rode with Joyce in her red convertible VW Beetle or walked the one mile to the embassy and then stopped at the fishmonger's, the greengrocer's and the bakery. By the time we finally walked toward home, Ginger's legs would be tired and she'd want to be carried. If I didn't comply, the African women who lived along our road scolded me, shouting and gesturing for me to pick her up.

The mountain air of Yaoundé summoned us out of doors for picnics with embassy personnel—the nurse, a secretary, and a couple of the marine security guards—or excursions with Joyce and the Bradley kids. We were finally settling into a life that resembled "normal."

# 5

# MARTIN

*While the children* and I were getting adjusted to life in Cameroon, Martin was often away helping Carl in Equatorial Guinea. Carl would later write a story about his friendship with Martin, a story that begins in Santa Isabel. Here is a bit of that story:

It was on the airport tarmac of a hot and humid African island located just three degrees north of the equator that I first saw Martin. He and his fellow passengers had just survived another flight on one of the two Convair 440s that comprised the world's newest airline of the world's newly independent state of Equatorial Guinea. I could never have known that the "Doc" walking toward the small terminal that day was one of the funniest people I've ever known and would become one of my greatest friends.

Fernando Po was a place of incredible beauty, with so many wonderful people, some very dangerous people and a few who could plot and carry out another person's death on a moment's notice. Into this place of perpetual intrigue, Martin Bradley, MD, walked toward the terminal as though he had not a thought or care in the world . . .

From that first evening on the island, I never tired of the sense of humor of this lanky guy from Pennsylvania. You never knew what he'd do next . . .

[He began by] planning the first "winter ski vacation" to ever be held on a tropical island. It involved asking some Swissaid workers to scrounge a travel film from Swiss Air, setting the room air conditioners to make it uncomfortably cold, planning an appropriate menu, and inviting guests who we knew, or thought we knew, had a sense of humor.

———➤

Seizing on the popularity of that evening's entertainment, Carl and Martin held frequent "meetings" of the Santa Isabel Ski Club.

Our family would often recall Martin's morale-boosting escapade and his many pranks over the years, including perhaps the most iconic. During Martin's 1970s days as an army colonel, on his hospital desk in Frankfurt sat a framed glossy of Gen. Omar Bradley (no relation). On the photo Martin had written, "Good luck, Son. You'll go far."

# 6

# KIND OF LIKE NORMAL

*Charles seemed to* like his kindergarten at the International School. Both he and Ginger enjoyed the hamburger/hot dog grill and the pool at the embassy's rec center. They were learning a little French by osmosis there in a Francophone country, and I was making a stab at it in French class. And Ginger's speech! I could only describe it as music—a melding of all the different speech sounds and patterns she'd been hearing: British English, Hausa, Spanish, French, Pidgin English, Pidgin French and native languages there in Cameroon.

We'd been evacuated on February 16, so an April 3, 1971, update to family was overdue:

> We were evacuated six weeks ago now, and the kids are finally beginning to calm down and stop yelling, "There's the police!" or "There's the Guardia!" every time they see a uniform. I do wonder if Ginger is taking her cue from Charles. When I tell people about Equatorial Guinea, they ask if I wasn't just absolutely terrified. But it's weird. I was tense for sure. I found that out on R and R. But there was just this strange feeling of life there not being real. I don't know if it will ever feel like it was real. Then too,

Mother, I guess I have some of your stoicism and a small smidgen of your faith. I can hear you quoting the scripture, "In nothing be anxious . . ."

I wrote you before about my friendship with Barbara, the Spanish ambassador's wife in Santa Isabel, and our mutual interest in art. Her husband tried to get permission from Macias for Barbara and me to visit the studio of a prominent Equatorial Guinean artist. Macias never relented. But then, guess what! After the kids and I arrived in Yaoundé the US Information Service Library here hosted an exhibit of the artist's work—and a personal appearance! I had to choke back the tears when I met him. I can't believe Macias allowed him out of the country!

I have two speech therapy clients now—embassy kids. It feels good to work in my profession. With such a big gap between finishing my M.A. and clinical fellowship year, and the time I'll be able to take my board exams, I'm excited to have this opportunity.

I'll try to give you a progress report from what Carl has told me of his work. Amazingly, despite the political violence, his program continues to be a success. His proposal for the next three phases of the smallpox/measles program was approved intact, much to everyone's surprise. The ambassador calls Carl the miracle worker, and Carl is glad he's making a real contribution to the implementation of our foreign policy. I've learned that's the purpose of AID, and the smallpox program is the only thing America has going in EG. The ambassador and the State Department don't want the program to go away, especially since the Russians, the Chinese and the North Koreans are gaining ground there every day. Two weeks ago the EG government asked Carl to vaccinate the entire population against cholera. Dr. Bradley from here in Yaoundé is over there helping. He and Carl say sticking needles in the Russian and Chinese communists was the most fun.

This assignment has been quite the experience for Carl. On about six occasions he has been left in charge of the embassy, sometimes for up to five days at a time. At what other post in the world would the smallpox-measles man ever serve as acting de facto chargé d'affaires? Rarely has anything come up that couldn't just wait until the chargé returned, but if anything should have happened— Carl was "it."

Well, I think that gets you up to date. At this point we don't really know about the future. Our chargé d'affaires wants Carl to take the Foreign Service Officer exam. He's considering it but also looking at other options.

Hopefully we'll soon have a date for our return home from this assignment. I'll keep you posted. Please write again soon. Can't wait to see you!

Big, big hugs to all of you,

Bee

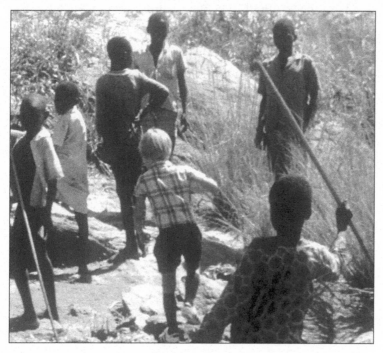

Charles with local boys, Cameroon, 1971

# 7

# THE ZOO

*The Volkswagen Beetle* skittered among the fissures and craters of the jungle road. Joyce Bradley and John, an English friend who accompanied us, traded off driving. I could have used experience at riding bucking broncos, because only the tightly wedged position of my children and me in the back seat kept us there.

It would take seven hours to cover the one hundred sixty miles from Yaoundé in Cameroon's highlands to the coast.

Despite the discomfort in getting there, our seaside rendezvous in the village of Victoria (now Limbe) was worth every mile. The children and I would spend Easter weekend with Carl, the first time together since our evacuation two months earlier, and Joyce would have the weekend with Martin.

Besides their activities in the smallpox/measles program, Martin and Carl had been working furiously to head off the cholera epidemic sweeping down the west coast of Africa toward Equatorial Guinea. After the weekend's respite in Victoria, they would have to go back into Macias country and continue the battle. Each one of us needed a calm and peaceful retreat.

When we finally arrived, I peeled myself, an inch at a time, out of the Beetle's back seat. There were hugs and excitement all around. Charles and Ginger were excited to see their dad, but without the Bradley children along they were soon ready for us to do something besides sit and talk. We promised that tomorrow we'd make a trip to the zoo recommended by the man at the hotel desk.

The next morning, I looked across the water toward Fernando Po, twenty miles away. Victoria sat at the foot of Mt. Cameroon, so if we happened to have a clear day, we would have a dramatic view of the island's volcanic peak, much like the view of Mt. Cameroon from the Bahia's terrace. Through the mist I could just make out a faint hint on the horizon, but nothing more.

After breakfast, Carl and I took the kids and left our bungalow to keep our promise. Just a short stroll. But the name zoo had given me the wrong idea of the attraction. We arrived at a lush tropical park tightly hugged by the jungle. No fence, gate or walkway interrupted the acres of grass. Banana trees, hardwood trees and vines complemented the delicate colors and aroma of orchids. I drank in the softness. And the quiet, broken only by the occasional song of an exotic bird, added to the morning's tranquility. There were no attendants and no other visitors. The stillness was complete. I let it soak in through every pore.

A sociable little monkey, a resident of the surrounding jungle no doubt, teased us. He'd join us for a while, scamper away, and then join us again.

Farther into the park, we came upon the first of eight or ten puny cages scattered over the expanse of green. They were rusted and had no safety rails. Concrete blocks under each corner elevated them about two feet, leaving mud and muck underneath.

Allow me to paint the scene of what happened next.

Our laughter splintered the quiet when we arrived at a cage housing two chimpanzees. Their chatter said, "Yay! We—have—company! Let us entertain you!" And we said, "You're so cute—and so funny!" There followed many minutes of mutual

merriment between human and chimp. An adult chimpanzee is
nearly six feet tall, and their reach is one and a half times their
height. Their shenanigans had our rapt attention.

"Oh look, Carl. There's our friendly monkey again," I said.
"He really likes Charles."

We all turned to watch the capers of our little escort. Charles
grinned. "Look, Mom. He's hanging on me." I snapped a picture
of the monkey hanging from Charles's shoulders.

Suddenly Ginger was screaming!

A chimp's long arms had reached through the bars. Two hands
gripped her neck and slammed the back of her head against the
cage.

We were screaming, shouting, screaming—all at once. It was
all confusion! You couldn't tell who was doing what!

"She's got her by the neck!"

The chimp lifted Ginger off the ground and swung her against
the iron bars. Kept swinging her—slamming her head against the
iron bars. Sharp, sawed-off, rusty iron bars.

"Carl, hurry!"

Sickening thud over and over as the chimp slammed her head
again.

Again and again.

Carl tried to free Ginger. "Move, Bee, I've got—"

The chimp knocked Carl down into the mud with one hand.
Her grip loosened on Ginger's neck.

She was holding her with just one hand now. Her attention
was diverted—this was our chance.

I reached down and pulled Ginger toward me.

She's free. Thank goodness, she's free.

Carl shouted, "Quick! Move her away!"

But the chimp grabbed my shoulders with both hands. Pain
seared as nails dug in. I was facing tree-trunk sized legs.

My face was heading toward the iron bars, but as Carl pulled himself from the mud, his movement distracted the chimp. My face was spared, but the grip on my shoulders didn't let up.

Carl's glasses were still in the mud, and he was blind without them. But he somehow—I've no idea how—pulled me free.

We all scrambled out of the chimp's reach. Stunned, we stood there. Just stood there. Staring. Silent, except for the sound of rapid, hard breathing.

Finally, the sight of blood running from Ginger's head snapped us from our trance. Carl stripped off his shirt to use as a compress. I fished Carl's glasses from the muck and wiped off what I could with the hem of my dress.

The attack chimp cowered in a far corner of the cage as the other shook a finger at her and screeched her reprimands. Our little monkey friend must have scampered back home to *his* mama, because he was nowhere in sight.

With no round of applause for the chimps, no standing ovation, no curtain calls, we trudged back to our bungalow in a half daze, Carl keeping the pressure on Ginger's bleeding head. When we got to our hotel, Dr. Joyce Bradley gave tetanus shots to Ginger and me. The scars on either side of Ginger's neck, and mine behind both shoulders, would be visible for two years, the reminder of our seaside respite.

―➤

When writing about this experience, I wondered whether the Victoria Zoo would still be there and whether it would have replaced those pitiful cages. I did some research. Yes. Current photos revealed a lovely park still as beautiful as I remembered. In 1993, conservation biologists concluded the zoo was the perfect place for their new wildlife center. Established initially as a sanctuary for rescued chimpanzees, their mission broadened to rescue, rehabilitation and reintroduction of rescued wildlife. The Limbe Wildlife Center is now the region's premier center for primate research.

When the center first opened, they had only one chimpanzee, Suzanne. She was the last resident of the former zoo. The age would be about right. I wonder.

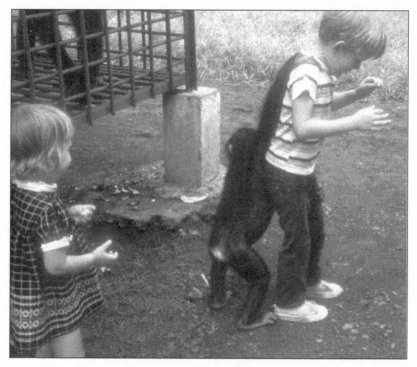

Just the second before—

# 8

# FRIENDLY FIRE

*Other than our* chimpanzee encounter, the seaside retreat had been both restful and energizing. But an event was about to happen that Ambassador Hoffacker would later cite as an example of the stress of life in Equatorial Guinea.

On April 11, Joyce and the children and I left Victoria to drive back to Yaoundé. Carl and Martin headed for Douala, where they would catch the little Convair for their twenty-minute flight back to Santa Isabel. Along with an Austrian gentleman from the International Monetary Fund, they were in the gate area when they saw another American who showed up in Santa Isabel off and on. I'll call him George. He and Carl exchanged their customary friendly banter. Once on board, Carl chose a front seat facing Martin and directly across the aisle from George. Carl had buckled his seatbelt in preparation for takeoff and held on his lap the diplomatic pouch handed to him in Douala.

Suddenly George bolted from his seat and lunged at Carl from across the aisle. He jerked Carl's glasses off and threw them to the floor, doubled up his fist and socked Carl on the left side of the face. He drew his arm back, preparing to hit Carl again, but Martin Bradley was on his feet. He moved between them and motioned for George to sit down. Returning to his seat, George said something like, "Bloeser, get out of here. You bother me." Martin escorted Carl, obviously stunned, to the back of the plane, checked his face and determined no special care was needed.

Before the brief flight landed, George walked to the back and offered a tearful apology. He said Carl had done nothing to trigger his attack.

Carl and Martin reported the event to Al Williams, and Al summoned George to his office. I don't know what was said except that George reiterated his apology. Reports all indicated the incident was out of character.

After this, he was seen wandering around the town carrying a plastic Virgin Mary statue and muttering to himself. I've never known what eventually happened to George.

# 9

# THE DAILIES

*I heard from* Carl. He reported these latest happenings in EG.

Beatings and missing persons are increasing. PNGs are routine.

After Macias nationalized the Hotel Bahia in February, he asked the woman comanager to stay on and manage the hotel as a government of Equatorial Guinea employee. She agreed, but after six weeks she couldn't take it anymore and decided to go home to Spain. Just before she was to leave, government officials detained her. Now she's being held until Macias decides whether he will allow her to leave the country.

The Russian, Chinese and North Korean embassies continue to grow while most others are dwindling. That's interesting, and I don't really understand it. If we can get by with two or three people in our embassy, why do the communist countries need so many people on staff? Al says they don't trust having any locals in their embassies—they bring in even their own housekeepers—whereas the US and others make it a point to give jobs to country nationals. The Swiss technical delegation families have gone, as well as families with various embassies. Even the diplomats from other African nations, except Guinea-Conakry, want to get out.

The Nigerian exodus continues despite efforts to frighten

them into staying. The GOEG tells them their countrymen who have returned home were killed as soon as they reached Nigeria. The Nigerians don't believe them and are leaving anyway. But they do face an uncertain future as their homeland begins to rebuild from the civil war. I wonder when Samuel will leave, and I wonder whether his home village is still standing. What has happened to his family there? Such heartache.

# 10

# CHANGING OF THE GUARD

*Many staff changes* occurred that winter and spring. Leonard Shurtleff succeeded Mike Hoyt as consul in Douala. Al and Carman
were transferred out of Equatorial Guinea on April 30, so Carl
would be working with a new team. Al was assigned as political
officer in the US embassy in Santa Domingo, Dominican Republic.

Carl had been furious with Al for not trying to stop the Guardia's invading our home when we unpacked our household
shipment, a day that now seemed so long ago. But over time he
realized confrontation was not a safe course, and he learned from
Al what should and what could be done in this type of environment. Just before the Williamses departed, Carl wrote a long letter
to Ambassador Hoffacker expressing wholehearted admiration.
He said the briefing at AID Washington emphasized the country
team concept and that in this smallest country team in the world,
Al Williams had made the concept a reality.

In pondering this quote from diplomat and historian George
Kennan's speech to fellow foreign service officers, I suppose our
family is fortunate Al was able to pull it off, even in Macias's
Equatorial Guinea:

What is important in the relations between two governments is not just, or predominantly, the what, but rather the how: the approach, the posture, the manner, the style of action. The most brilliant undertaking can be turned into a failure if it is clumsily and tactlessly executed. There are, on the other hand, few blunders which cannot be survived, if not redeemed, when matters are conducted with grace and with feeling.

Before Al left, he reported that Macias closed more schools, which were already barely functioning due to the departure of all the Spanish teachers and administrators. No locals were available to teach because those educated beyond eighth grade were dead, in prison or had fled the country.

On May 7, 1971, one week after Al and Carman's departure, Macias canceled all key elements of the constitution and assumed "all direct powers of Government and Institutions . . ." In other words, all powers of the executive, legislative and judicial branches of government, as well as those of the Council of the Republic that had been established to control the executive. Macias was officially now the potentate.

—→

For the Association for Diplomatic Studies and Training's Moments in Diplomatic History project, Ambassador Hoffacker would later say: "As early as March 1969, Newsweek reported that in only a few months after independence, the Macias government had brought the country to the verge of ruin . . . . The treasury was empty. The cabinet was rent by violent quarrels. . . . His foreign minister and UN representative were beaten to death."

Africa expert Randall Fegley said, "Macias was a maniac with a record of corruption, sadism and psychiatric disorders. . . . Proportionally his rule equaled that in Nazi-occupied Europe in terms of brutality."

A French writer, Rene Pelissier, said, "Nowhere else in modern times had a tyrant of Macias' magnitude managed to destroy his country and annihilate his own people so extensively and persistently. . . ."

Into this environment, following a woefully inadequate review of their histories and personnel files, State replaced Al and Carman with Al Erdos as chargé d'affaires and Don Leahy as administrative officer.

# 11

# COLD WAR DECISION MAKING

*By May 30*, 1971, memo and cable traffic had been heavy for six weeks among key decision makers: Ambassador Hoffacker, CDC, USAID regional office, USAID Washington—and Carl. They argued the pros and cons of Carl's leaving Equatorial Guinea June 20 rather than September 20, his contract end date, and whether a replacement would be assigned.

Carl emphasized his willingness to abide by the joint decision but also his strong preference for a June 20 departure because of the hardship imposed by our family separation.

CDC laid out the arguments on both sides but awaited USAID's pending decision regarding the end date of the entire West and Central Africa program. There'd been no new smallpox cases for nearly a year, but CDC believed it was too soon to stop surveillance activities. And they still hoped to gain better control of measles."

Our program in Equatorial Guinea was particularly on the USAID chopping block. In Washington's cutbacks they saw limited benefit of continuing aid, given the difficulty of working with Macias and his government.

Ambassador Hoffacker argued from a Cold War perspective. He "absolutely did not agree" (reported by Jean Roy after his discussion with the ambassador) with USAID's desire to end the program. He wanted it to continue, with Carl if possible, or with a replacement if necessary. He argued its heightened importance in the East-West power struggle at a time when communist influence was gaining momentum and America's decreasing daily. Carl had maintained a fruitful relationship with Macias's government and a friendly US posture in a deteriorating political and economic reality. The ambassador emphasized the smallpox/measles program was 100 percent of the USAID presence there and was appreciated throughout the country. (Ambassador Hoffacker still called Carl "the miracle worker.")

As the debate continued, Carl argued that USAID's pulling out just when GOEG had approved his proposal for the next three phases of the program—and amazingly, approved it intact—would create more enemies. It would foster greater distrust of America than already existed.

In the end, all parties came to a joint decision to release Carl June 20 due to the unusual political and family circumstances. The Public Health Service would post Carl back in the States. CDC would send another operations officer to Equatorial Guinea to fill the gap until the end date of the entire West Africa program. Ambassador Hoffacker said he would write CDC on this decision and related matters.

Just weeks in the future, the question of a continued CDC/USAID presence would become a moot point.

# 12

# SO LONG, FAREWELL

*On June 16,* 1971, four months after we were evacuated, Charles, Ginger and I flew back to Santa Isabel to pack up the house for our family's final departure from Equatorial Guinea.

Loyal Samuel had remained there for Carl for the four months the children and I were in Cameroon. Now as he helped me pack, he forced a smile, but his eyes sometimes glistened with tears. I worried about Samuel, this precious man who had defied the Guardia, risking his life for us. When we left Nigeria, we'd helped our staff find other employers. But here, people who would have hired household help were fleeing. I would never know whether Samuel made it back to his homeland.

With three days to pack, I gave linens and pots and pans to Samuel for him to use or to pass on and gave toys and children's clothes to the neighborhood playmates. (Charles was able to have some playtime with his friends and, fortunately, didn't see any Guardia or police.)

We had a parting glimpse of Caesar, that lion-looking cat who had caused such alarm at the airport the year before but hadn't been seen since the day we were evacuated. Samuel had tried and failed to lure him with food. A couple of days after we returned, Caesar appeared up under the eaves of the house. He had grown feral. He stared at us without recognition, did not react to our calls and soon disappeared back into the crawlspace under the roof.

Carl sent a final report to Macias's minister of health, outlining what had been accomplished. He stressed the country now had a method of disease control for attacking several other communicable diseases.

And Carl had a few final days to work with his right-hand man. This young man, whom I've called Ricardo, did a stellar job as Carl's administrative assistant and had become a good friend. He was from an old influential Fernandino family, with several of his ancestors listed on any site of prominent names in the history of Fernando Po. Ricardo's beloved grandmother had been an avid stamp collector, and Ricardo had inherited her three bulging albums with stamps from all over the world. He wanted Carl to have them, and we were both touched by his gift.

Our embassy's new chargé, Al Erdos, hosted a farewell reception for us on June 18 at the American residence and invited the diplomatic community. He sent a special request to the minister of foreign affairs. (And who might that be? Of course it was President Macias. He had added that role to his portfolio after the death—murder?—of the previous minister.) The request to *Excelentisimo Señor Ministro* asked permission for the embassy to invite members of the Equatorial Guinean government and friends from the Organization of African Unity, "if the ministry perceives no objection." Several were allowed to attend.

High regard for Carl and his work was apparent at the reception. And besides the many expressions of gratitude, he received a good-bye present from the Russian Nicolay Ivanov—a bottle of Russian vodka.

Just before Al Williams transferred to Santo Domingo, he had written a lengthy letter to CDC Director Dr. David Sencer. In addition to many other laudatory remarks, he said about Carl:

On his eventual departure from this assignment, his legacy will be a confident and trained Guinean medical infrastructure capable of carrying out a continuing program of activities related to communicable disease, a rare if highly sought-after achievement in this part of the world.

Carl and everyone in the smallpox program could be justifiably proud. West Africa had the highest smallpox rates per thousand in the world at the outset of the campaign in 1967 and was projected to be the toughest place for program success. It had the poorest health and communication infrastructure. Problems of transportation and terrain were constant. Tribal rivalries and conflicts and political instability and war became familiar.

But even with civil war and a thousand large and small hurdles, more than 153 million smallpox vaccinations and more than 28 million measles vaccinations were administered in the region. Months of continued surveillance in every nomad encampment, teaming marketplace, and all-but-inaccessible pockets of the rainforests would determine that transmission of smallpox in the entire region had been stopped with that May 1970 case in Nigeria.

The five-year goal of eradicating smallpox in West and Central Africa was completed early—in three and a half years and sixteen million dollars under budget.

# 13

# AND THEN THERE WERE FIVE

*Besides the formal* reception for us, the embassy hosted an intimate casual evening with just the Americans. Dinner and the monthly movie newly arrived on the government circuit—*The Dirty Dozen*, I think. With our departure, there would be only five in the American community—the new chargé, his wife and son, and the new administrative officer and his wife.

Chargé d'Affaires Alfred Erdos, the son of parents who had immigrated to America from Hungary, was over six feet tall and burly. His wife, Jean, didn't seem nurturing like Ambassador Hoffacker's wife, Connie, or playful like Carman, but she was gracious—a dignified professional woman. Her running of the American residence would be more formal than Carman's for sure. Their son, Christopher, two years old and all decked out in short pants, knee-high stockings, fancy suit jacket and a ruffled shirt, stayed close to his mother.

Don Leahy, the quiet new administrative officer, was short and slight of build. Erdos would later say, "Don was half my size." I took an immediate liking to Rosita Leahy, a gentle, sweet-tempered lady from Quito, Ecuador.

But something was wrong. At dinner and throughout the evening, in speech, facial expression and bearing, Chargé Erdos made it clear. He was top dog. And an angry one. He snapped at Don Leahy in front of everyone.

"Don, do this."

"Don't do that!"

"You can never even thread the projector!"

Don endured the censure in silence.

On the way back to our house at the end of the evening, Carl said, "Erdos always flies off the handle. You'd think he was Don's drill sergeant." Carl's work had been increasingly on the island, as vaccination was completed on the mainland, so he had had two and a half months to observe the working relationship between Leahy and Erdos. Once Al and Carman left, almost two months ago now, the dynamic between the two men emerged and became increasingly pronounced.

In the stress of Equatorial Guinea, often referred to as the worst post in the foreign service, only a charitable and supportive relationship between the two American families would enable them to function. Except for the episode with our shipment in which Carl fumed at Al, we had a warm relationship with him and Carman. They included us in everything possible, and the tensions of Equatorial Guinea drove us closer. Even with that support, this post exacted a price our family would have preferred not to pay.

I worried about the four adults and about Christopher even more. Would he go to bed hearing screams from the police station? What twists and turns would affect Christopher's young life before the Erdos family left this post?

On June 20, our family flew out of Santa Isabel for the last time on the weekly Iberia flight to Madrid. We would have preferred to stay in West Africa—in a different country. But smallpox had been eradicated here and the entire program would soon be phasing out. For now, we were returning to a public health posting in the States. Dallas, Texas.

As the plane pulled onto the runway, I was bathed in an enormous wave of relief. We were escaping the snake pit, thankful to leave the deadly vipers in power far behind. Sadly, we were also leaving their victims behind. The people enclosed in the rain forest's deceptive beauty had no option to escape, and we were powerless to intervene.

Outside the terminal, Al Erdos and Don Leahy waved good-bye.

# 14

# ROUGH REENTRY

*Carl had much-needed* leave time coming. After a week in Spain and Portugal, we stopped in Santo Domingo to spend a few days with Al and Carman. (We would later host them for several days in Texas.) The first thing Al wanted to hear was news of how the embassy had functioned in the two months since his departure.

"So how are Erdos and Leahy getting along?"

Carl said, "Well, I guess they'll be okay if they don't kill each other first."

When Al and Carman were free that week, Carl updated Al, and we all reminisced about what we had lived through. Some of those recollections had us in stitches. With others, we were amazed we had gotten out alive.

After those few days with our embassy "family," we had a two-day visit in Haiti, which shares the island with the Dominican Republic. Then the last leg of our journey "home."

On our first morning back in America, we left the hotel room and went downstairs to the coffee shop. We were looking at the menu when Charles looked up and saw an African American employee clearing the table next to ours. His eyes brightened and his face lit up with a big grin as he shouted, "How did *he* get here?"

Reunions with family and friends nurtured us, like being wrapped in a warm, familiar blanket. These were the welcome, comfortable things. The joyous things. And we began, a bit timidly at first, to reconnect with our church family.

But reverse culture shock lurked around every corner. Painful. People were too soft. Choices too numerous and overwhelming. Fifteen different kinds of deodorant or toothpaste or detergent was ridiculous. And tedious. Did we really need an entire grocery aisle for different kinds of cereal? What a consuming, throwaway society!

As I opened accounts at the bank, the electric company and the phone company, I had to supply our previous address. Every employee made a face. "Africa? Ew! I betcha sure are glad to be back home!" In high dudgeon, internally, I pasted on a semi-polite quizzical look.

*Let's see now, let me try on that "representation" look.*

Despite everything that had happened, despite Macias, we loved Africa, and we loved the people we'd gotten to know. Did people in the States have no interest in anyone outside themselves—ourselves?

Social interactions were the worst. I faked civility at what I perceived as upside down values all around me. You don't like your sofa? So what? Your stove is on the blink? That's nothing! Do you hear—nothing! None of this is important! Don't you get it? It's. Not. Im-por-tant! Do you have to walk an hour each way to haul home a bucket of water, and unsafe water at that?

Our experiences put material goods in perspective. One of my guiding scriptures says, "But godliness with contentment is great gain. For we brought nothing into the world, and we can take nothing out of it. But if we have food and clothing, we will be content with that." (I Timothy 6:6–8, NIV)

It was hard to make friends. Hard to find common interests, common concerns. "How 'bout those Cowboys?" We had left Africa, but Africa wouldn't leave us. We cornered anyone who gave us a hint of an opening and tried to share the realities of life outside our borders. After the first five minutes of surface curiosity, our captives' expressions glazed over and they eyed the nearest exit, except for the few who hungered to hear more and the still rarer person who asked to see our slides.

I soon learned not to talk about Africa. It was not a topic with which others could connect. I got quiet because our African experience occupied all the large and small spaces in my mind. In my heart.

As it is in grieving the death of a spouse or a child, so it is for the person surviving a tornado or the person who has witnessed great human tragedy. Friends are ready for you to get back to normal long before you are able.

But there was one question I still pondered. Why did Al and Ambassador Hoffacker encourage Carl to bring us to Equatorial Guinea when they knew so much about the horror of it? I've finally learned what I think is the answer—their perspectives as career foreign service officers. It was part of the job. Both had been in situations where bullets were flying all around them. My perspective was small town. It was healthcare. It was sheltered minister's daughter. And I do think that as things deteriorated, Al's approach kept us as safe as we could possibly have been.

In Dallas, we helped our children fit into their new surroundings. For three-year-old Ginger, all was smooth sailing.

Charles constructed ever more elaborate structures and scenes, often incorporating Ginger in his scenes. And any time he could gather several other children, he led them in a running parade, he as the bearer of the American flag.

He came home from first grade saying he didn't like his school.

When I asked why, he said, "Everybody is just plain white." Yes, there were things he missed.

But we soon found that the trauma Charles had heard about and experienced brought difficult memories. He was anxious—always looking over his shoulder, having nightmares on occasion. His drawings turned dark, pages and pages of thick black lines with sharp angles. Rifles, knives and bayonets dominated the scenes. It hurt our hearts, and like any parents we asked ourselves what we could have done to shield him. Many of the pictures felt so disturbing I would later decide to get rid of them.

While we were away in Africa, a good friend from my grad school days had gone on to complete her doctorate in psychology. Now she gave invaluable information and support in dealing with traumatic experiences. Charles made friends, and his nightmares and knife-filled drawings decreased.

Despite the negative aspects of his experience in Equatorial Guinea, Charles's empathy for his friends and their situation there would become a lifelong compassion for those suffering poverty or violence.

Ginger, three years younger, had had quite a different set of experiences. Even these many years later, she remembers kindness and affection from our African household staff. She recalls being carried, cared for and protected by them, a protection she grieves we were unable to offer in return. And to her mind Carl and I were calm and confident, even in Equatorial Guinea. She doesn't remember ever sensing danger.

As for Carl and me, we never got past the longing for that small tribe of people with the common bond of having served in the developing world. People among whom so much of wonder, so much of pathos, so much of horror can be shared, even when unspoken.

Even though we were not diplomats, a quote from George

Kennan's address to fellow foreign service officers seems to apply:

> To some extent, I fear, the professional diplomatist will always remain in his own country and particularly in this one a person apart, the bearer of a view of the outside world which his fellow citizens cannot entirely follow and a view of his own country, while it does not cause him to love it the less, causes him to see it in other ways than his neighbors at home can ever be expected to see it.

# 15

## SHOCK WAVE

*It was a* Wednesday afternoon. We'd been back in the States six weeks. Just home from work, Carl sat at the table and opened the afternoon paper.

US Diplomat's Death Probed—2nd Found Deranged

SANTA ISABEL, Equatorial Guinea (UPI)—US diplomats today began an investigation of the death of an American foreign service officer and the apparent mental collapse of another in this steaming island capital off the coast of West Africa.

The diplomats said the body of Donald J. Leahy, 47, was found when they arrived to investigate what the State Department called confusing reports from the scene.

They also found another American official, Alfred J. Erdos, 46, and said he was "incapacitated and apparently suffering from a mental breakdown." He too was in the chancery. . . .

Reports from Madrid said Lewis Hoffacker, US ambassador to the Cameroon and Equatorial Guinea, was cutting short a home leave and flying back to Africa. The

Spanish reports said the situation was confused but the situation was caused "by personal problems between employees.". . . (September 1, 1971, *Dallas Times Herald*)

Horror and grief grabbed hold and would not let go. Our phone stayed busy all evening with calls to and from family, friends and colleagues.

US Diplomat's Death in Africa Laid to Violence

The unexplained death of American diplomat Donald J. Leahy at a two-man post in the island capital of Equatorial Guinea appears to be "the result of violence," the State Department said yesterday. . . . (Thursday, September 2, 1971, *The Washington Post*, United Press International)

Articles peppered news outlets for the next several days. They delivered speculation along with the few known facts as they described a macabre murder scene. Don's body had been found stabbed repeatedly with a long pair of scissors.

Facts reached us from those who found the body within a few hours of the murder—in the office Carl had so recently vacated. That Al Erdos murdered Don Leahy was never in question, was never denied. I share here information from my notes of a phone conversation with Don Leahy's widow, Rosita, a letter from Rosita, and official State Department reports about the events of August 30, 1971.

For an unknown length of time after he murdered Don Leahy, Al Erdos remained alone inside the embassy with the body and with the door bolted. The consul from Douala, Cameroon, Leonard Shurtleff, rushed to Santa Isabel by charter flight. He had been dispatched to investigate strange and disturbing reports received that afternoon from Erdos after earlier transmissions from Don Leahy over a radio located in the chancery vault. When Shurtleff arrived by taxi from the airport, Erdos refused to open the door, saying he would speak only to Ambassador Hoffacker. But the ambassador was in the United States on home leave. Shurtleff spent some time then on foot and by telephone trying to locate Erdos's wife, Jean. He first walked to the residence. The staff told him Jean had taken Christopher and gone to the Cameroonian ambassador's residence.

In a letter to Carl and me dated September 30, 1971, one month after her husband was murdered, and later through her sobs in a telephone conversation, Rosita Leahy told us her memory of the heartbreaking story from that point on. Shurtleff came to the Leahys' house looking for Don. When he found Don not there, he asked if Rosita could show him the way to the Cameroonian residence. They walked there together.

Rosita said apparently while Erdos remained locked inside the embassy, he had phoned his wife and instructed her to go to the Cameroonian residence. Rosita heard from someone that Jean had sought asylum, but that the Cameroonian chargé refused because he didn't want to take responsibility for such a decision in the absence of his ambassador. Rosita didn't know whether this was true.

Having finally located Jean Erdos, Shurtleff, Rosita, and Jean, with Christopher, walked to the US chancery. They arrived there about six-thirty in the evening. Erdos said he wanted to speak to his wife alone, so Jean entered, carrying Christopher, and the door was again locked.

Rosita wrote that she and Shurtleff put their ears to the heavy door, unsuccessfully trying to hear what was said inside. Shurtleff then left to use the phone at a nearby bar. Soon the Nigerian ambassador, Wellington Bassey, the ranking member of the diplomatic corps in Santa Isabel, arrived in his embassy's Mercedes and parked out front. By this time a crowd, including local police, had begun to gather outside even though there were no sounds and no clues as to what was going on.

Jean, who had done legal work for the State Department until recently, and Al Erdos had been alone in the chancery for about an hour when Jean came out for a moment and told Shurtleff her husband was out of control. She then stepped back inside, and in a minute or two Alfred Erdos, Jean and Christopher left the chancery and were escorted to the Nigerian embassy car.

Rosita's letter said, "Erdos . . . was walking out of the embassy, under security, and yet without us knowing what he had done inside, [he was] speaking cordially to the sizeable crowd that had gathered outside . . ."

Shurtleff later reported in his detailed account in the Foreign Service Journal that as the family walked to the waiting car, Erdos pulled him aside and said, "I lost my cool. I killed Don."

Rosita said the Nigerian ambassador sped away with the family. (He would give the family asylum until the US State Department could negotiate getting them out of the country.)

Rosita reported she and Shurtleff dashed into the embassy through a large pool of blood just inside the front door. As Shurtleff rushed through the bloody scene in the reception area and hurriedly searched the Leahy and Erdos offices and the vault, Rosita Leahy opened the door to Carl's former office, where she discovered the savagely murdered body of her husband.

"The doors had been locked, and for what we saw inside the chancery, he must have tried to open the door and get out, but this Erdos dragged him back to your office, where we found my Don."

Shurtleff's official reports say Don had been gagged and bound and had been stabbed numerous times. Evidence indicated the attack began inside the vault near one of the radios. Blood-soaked floors, clothing and papers, and blood-smeared walls fouled much of the reception area, offices and vault. One of the wounds had nicked the jugular.

The greatest amount of blood was on and near the front door, where Don had apparently made a final attempt to escape.

After the deed was done, as Erdos's words were later transcribed from court testimony, "I looked, and the whole embassy was just a gory mess, blood just over the place, indescribable, and I thought, *What is this? Not all of that can come from the human body.*"

Evidence indicated Erdos dragged Don's body into Carl's office, where Rosita made the horrifying discovery. A smallpox/measles program binder sat neatly on the desk awaiting Carl's replacement.

These and many other details are known about the chilling event of August 30, but questions remain that will never be answered.

Prior history about Erdos was mixed, and much of it not known to those making the decision to assign him to Equatorial Guinea. A few individuals who served under Erdos at prior embassy posts had remained silent as long as Erdos could affect their careers. They were silent too long for Don Leahy.

As I grieved I wrestled with uncomfortable thoughts. Would Carl's presence have kept the situation between the two men from going critical? Would Don still be alive if we had not left Africa ahead of schedule? I remembered Carl's eerily prescient comment: "I guess they'll be okay if they don't kill each other first."

Attorney Aubrey Daniel had made his fame with his successful prosecution in the Mÿ Lai massacre case. He now defended

Erdos in the five-day trial in an Alexandria, Virginia, federal district court. The defense team operated on a theory that Erdos was in a paranoid psychotic episode brought on by living in Equatorial Guinea. Erdos claimed the stressors such as constant surveillance of diplomats' homes and offices and the sound of screams coming from the police station across the street from the residence had driven him over the edge. Someone who attended the trial told us that one thing brought up as an example of life there was the attempted arrest of our six-year-old son.

Carl, the only person who had witnessed the two-man working relationship between Erdos and Leahy, offered to testify. We went to Washington and stayed there for the duration of the trial because Carl was determined to be available in case they made a last-minute decision to call him. They did not.

The defense had summoned our unruffled, take-everything-in-stride chargé Al Williams to testify, and he flew in from Santo Domingo. But once the defense learned Al had, in fact, requested to extend his Santa Isabel posting for another year, the defense did not put him on the stand. But I will always wonder why the prosecution did not call him or Carl.

The jury sided with the prosecution view that Erdos was feigning insanity. On March 3, 1972, after deliberating for two and a half hours, they returned a conviction of voluntary manslaughter. The judge sentenced Erdos to ten years in prison. He served about three, from November 8, 1973, until his parole in late 1976.

Consul Len Shurtleff, the first person after Rosita to see Leahy's body, said the State Department implicitly accepted and supported the insanity defense. It granted Erdos full disability retirement with pension, even before the trial. After the murder, State closed the US embassy in Santa Isabel. According to diplomats' reports, for the next seven years the United States government sent no American to live in Equatorial Guinea.

# 16

# A GRIEF ACROSS THE OCEAN

*October 13, 1971,* Wednesday evening.

We might have been finished in Equatorial Guinea, but its bottomless pit of sorrow was not finished with us. Prior to the trial, Jean Erdos telephoned from her temporary apartment in Washington, DC. Her husband had entered psychiatric treatment at George Washington University Medical Center on his arrival on US soil.

Jean said we would want to know what had happened to the Equatorial Guinean nationals who worked for us. She talked with me for a while and then with Carl. The following is taken directly from the notes I wrote during Jean's conversation with me, and is as close to her exact wording as I could record. I have chosen not to reveal names of any Guinean who worked for us.

About the middle of August, a great deal of harassment of the US embassy began. Jean thought all of this was what brought on "the tragedy."

First our embassy driver and our courier were arrested. The police brought the driver by the embassy to get his pay and said they were deporting him to Bata. (This fit with Macias's practice of imprisoning people from the island in the Bata Jail and people from the mainland in Black Beach Prison on the island, essentially preventing families from bring them food and comfort.)

Carl's administrative assistant and friend, Ricardo, had worked with both the smallpox program and the embassy after our departure. Jean said he was in Bata when the harassment started and never came back. The embassy assumed he had been arrested over there, and they soon received confirmation. Another diplomat told them an employee of his had been at the six-room hotel in Bata and had seen the authorities drag Ricardo out of his room in his pajamas in the middle of the night, arrest him and, there in the hallway, beat him severely. The officers dragged him away, and he was not seen again. How to shake this grief over the suffering of such a dear friend, a kind and gentle man, and loyal coworker? Thoughts of what was done to him after the beating in the hotel are too awful to ponder.

Many Spaniards had been arrested and were in Black Beach Prison. One was beaten "almost to a pulp." Jean said they thought the man was suffering from brain damage. Someone later saw the man on the infamous grass-cutting (with scissors) crew out by the airport for a while, and others later saw him back at Black Beach.

Someone also saw another of our employees in Black Beach.

Shortly after the arrest of all these people, the Americans and Spaniards were told their safety could no longer be guaranteed outside the city limits of Santa Isabel. Travel down the coast or up to the mountain without special permission from the president had already been prohibited.

About the same time, Dr. Watson, Equatorial Guinea's ambassador to Cameroon, was arrested and held in Black Beach prison. Someone, Jean didn't remember who, saw them take Ambassador Watson from there and put him on a boat for Bata.

Jean said no employees of other embassies were harassed, except for the arrest of the driver for the Ghanaian embassy right after he delivered a note to our embassy. But what about Samuel? And what about Sunday and Friday?

Jean continued, "We couldn't figure out why the Americans had been singled out for this treatment, as we had no stake. Apparently, the president [Macias] thought Americans were involved in a plot against him. We heard that one or more of our employees who had been arrested signed a statement to that effect. I wouldn't be surprised if they had, under the circumstances. And I wouldn't blame them."

Ambassador Hoffacker later reported that Ambassador Watson "had died under grisly torture and may have implicated the United States in some kind of plot."

On the Saturday before the "tragic Monday," Elame Munge, the Ghanaian chargé d'affaires, had been at the residence for dinner and tried to persuade Erdos to visit the families of the employees who had worked for the Americans. Erdos responded he was concerned more than he could say, but he felt any overtures he might make to the families would only endanger them.

Jean continued, "Lots of people were being arrested at that time. We saw much of the brutality going on across the street at the police station. People were being beaten with clubs in the booking area right behind the main gate. One time a police van pulled up, and they pulled a body out of the back, just like a carcass of meat, and threw it on the ground. It was all too much. We commented many times that we were glad you were out of there. The arrest of the employees would be even more upsetting to you since you had worked with them much longer." How right she was. How powerless we all were to protect those who'd served us so faithfully.

Then Jean shared the news that the baby of my friends from the Ghanaian embassy had died following convulsions and horrible malpractice at the local hospital. Jean said she knew I would want to know. So much tragic loss. I handed the phone to Carl.

I knew that after the embassy was closed, Samuel, Sunday and Friday would have been out of work, and worse, no longer protected by the embassy. If others who worked for the Americans had been arrested, what chance did they have? And they'd been resented by other Nigerians because of their employment with the embassy. Where could they go? Or hide? I clung to a thin sliver of hope they had escaped—somehow.

I found myself crying easily for months after all this.

Erdos died in 1983 of a heart attack at age fifty-eight. His obituary in the magazine *State* made no mention of his manslaughter conviction. Lewis Hoffacker and Leonard Shurtleff, who both retired as ambassadors, are deceased. Jean Erdos and Rosita Leahy are also deceased.

# 17

# IS A PUZZLEMENT

*As I researched* published material for this memoir, it pleased me to see several historians include mention of Carl's program in Equatorial Guinea in their histories, even though Carl isn't named.

Randall Fegley said in *Equatorial Guinea: An African Tragedy* that the one thing USAID sponsored in Equatorial Guinea was a "successful campaign against smallpox and measles" that "covered the whole of the country."

Suzanne Cronjé, in *Equatorial Guinea—The Forgotten Dictatorship: Forced Labour and Political Murder in Central Africa,* published by the Anti-Slavery Society, mentioned that America had given some assistance, "for instance, a mass campaign against smallpox and measles carried out with US/AID help . . ."

It was hard to believe we'd been there, that we actually lived in Equatorial Guinea, lived that experience. But in case my memory had played tricks on me, I had proof in a drawerful of cables and letters.

First, there's the March 11, 1970 letter from the CDC (then called the NCDC) security representative confirming Carl's top-secret security clearance to serve in the "critical-sensitive position" in Equatorial Guinea. This document was copied to the doctor who was then director of the Smallpox Eradication Program (SEP), NCDC, the program management officer and assistant director, SEP, NCDC, and the administrative officer, SEP, Atlanta. Then there are Carl's monthly activity reports to CDC.

One of the letters in my files is from Al Williams to Dr. David Sencer, director of CDC. Al wrote the two packed-full pages on April 12, 1971, shortly before he left Africa. The first page commended Carl's work in the smallpox/measles program in Equatorial Guinea. Carl was a skillful negotiator, Al said, even dealing effectively with a minister of health known to be unfriendly to the West.

Then came another full page praising Carl's contributions. He said that Carl, as "50% of the US Government establishment in Equatorial Guinea," had been called on to handle functions normally assigned to State Department personnel.

Al talked about Carl's "keen political awareness and sensitivity . . . work in a hostile environment with maximum effectiveness . . . contribution to the smooth functioning of this Embassy both on administrative and substantive matters."

He concluded that, "Indeed, during my occasional absences, I have felt no compunctions about leaving him as the acting de facto chargé d'affaires. . . . In short, Mr. Bloeser has been a definite asset to this Embassy and has contributed immeasurably to promoting a favorable image of official American representation in this country."

In the May 6, 1971, response, Dr. Bill Foege, director of the Smallpox Eradication Program at CDC, thanked the chargé d'affaires for his letter to Dr. Sencer, and said:

"While we are proud of the West African Smallpox Eradication/Measles Control Program and of the individuals involved in the program, it is particularly gratifying to have you take the time to focus on an individual who deserves special recognition."

Ambassador Hoffacker's May 31, 1971, handwritten draft cable to CDC concludes with, "I shall write to Dr. Foege on this and related matters, including our continued high regard for Bloeser's performance."

A March 28, 2014, email from Al Williams to me, after Carl's passing, said:

> My thoughts often drift back to our days together in Equatorial Guinea when we all shared such an intense several years in that country. My memories of that post remain vivid to this day, sometimes evoking smiles and at other times relief that we all left alive. Few people in our respective professions have had the opportunity to experience what you, Carl, and I lived through . . .

So I puzzle over this statement on page 47 of the book *CDC and the Smallpox Crusade*, published by CDC:

"Also, the twentieth and last country added to the smallpox eradication program, Equatorial Guinea, is not discussed in this account. OCEAC provided supplies, equipment, and administrative and surveillance assistance to Equatorial Guinea, but neither CDC staff nor other US personnel had a direct role in the eradication program there."

# 18

## *THE DOGS OF WAR* AND THE LONG SHADOW OF MACIAS

*When the phone* rang that afternoon in 1974, I was surprised to hear J. Grant Burke on the other end of the line. I hadn't talked to Grant since the day, two weeks after my arrival in Santa Isabel, when Carman's startling note was taped on our door and he had been PNG'd. Grant and Carl had spoken several times after the murder and during the trial. He had also written Carl a couple of years ago with disturbing news. The *International Herald-Tribune*'s Paris edition reported Macias had shot fifty rioting Nigerians from his new Russian armored car. Again, my persistent concern. What about Samuel?

Now Grant sounded fired up about something! I handed the phone to Carl.

"Go out this minute and buy Forsyth's new novel, *The Dogs of War*. You'll recognize every person, every detail. It's Equatorial Guinea! It's unbelievable."

By now we were living next door to the US Indian Health Service hospital in Sacaton, Arizona, where Carl was hospital administrator. We immediately drove to the nearest bookstore. Frederick Forsyth had been one of Carl's favorite authors since *The Day of the Jackal* and *The Odessa File*. (Carl would later adopt

*The Shepherd* as essential reading at Christmas.) Now we plunged into *The Dogs of War*, where Macias's shadow still followed us. Would we ever leave that surreal life behind?

We accepted as fiction the novel's account of all the preparations—how the mercenaries were hired, how the ship was acquired and outfitted, how weapons were secretly purchased from arms dealers. But the target country! Zangaro! Forsyth employed only a thin disguise of his setting—the fictional mineral-rich mountain that provided the motivation for the plot, and the two sections of Zangaro separated by a wide river rather than the island-mainland divide. But this could not deceive a reader who had lived there. Not with the dozens of recognizable identifying details.

In the most minute particulars, the novel matched Macias himself, key cabinet ministers, specific murders of those ministers and the means of their execution, the rusty weapons, the shape and dimensions of the harbor, and details of the country's two airplanes. I was floored. "Oh my goodness, Carl. He's even got the little Convair 440s and their exact flight schedule!" Carl remarked on Forsythe's precision in describing the mercenaries' landing spot hidden from palace view at the bottom of the harbor cliff. All so close to our house! As the main character, Cat Shannon, prowled the streets, reconnoitering, I could just see him walk from the palace plaza the one block over and three blocks up. Did he pause just a moment in front of our house?

In the past we had told people to read Graham Greene's book about Haiti, *The Comedians,* to get a feel for what it was like in Equatorial Guinea. Now we said, "Read *The Dogs of War*. It's not *like* Equatorial Guinea. It *is* Equatorial Guinea."

In the coming weeks, people in our little circle from EG days read the novel, reread it and phoned back and forth, talking about the spot-on accuracy. We speculated as to who would have—could have—supplied Forsyth with such precise detail. Carl and others thought there were only three possible sources and were almost certain they knew which person it was. The country was isolated and unknown. No one who had lived there was writing about the place. Journalists were banned. And Spain prohibited any mention of her former colony in the press, made it a violation of the official Secrets Act. Forsythe had to have an inside source. We'd never know for sure who.

In 1977, three years after *The Dogs of War* was published, Carl was working in preventive medicine in Saudi Arabia. One day, he rushed in the door, waving a scrap of newspaper. "Look at this!" He handed me the clipping, which was, to the best of my memory, not more than a couple of column inches. Carl saved a lot of news clippings and always wrote on them the publication's name and the date. I am sure the clipping went into his collection, but I haven't been able to locate it.

I remember the item being about a mercenary who had been arrested, on some rather minor charge I think. In the course of the questioning, he claimed Forsyth had hired him and other mercenaries to pull off the coup described in *The Dogs of War*. He further claimed they had been on their way to Equatorial Guinea but were arrested at the port in the Canary Islands.

I was stunned. "What if it had come off while we were there! Four blocks from our house!" That long shadow of Macias gave me the shivers.

We didn't see or hear anything relating to that little news item over the coming months. But in March 1978, after another mercenary's gun battle with police in England ended in his suicide, the *London Sunday Times* came into possession of his diary. A mercenary keeping a diary? Surprising. Entries in the diary claimed knowledge of Forsyth's involvement in the attempted coup.

Forsyth denied the entire story. He dismissed it, saying the paper "added two plus two and got seventy-three." The *Times* continued to investigate, but we heard nothing further, neither then nor two years later when the movie based on the book was released.

But the matter wouldn't rest there. In 2005, Adam Roberts, staff writer for *The Economist* and then Johannesburg bureau chief, was doing research for his book *The Wonga Coup*, about the 2004 attempt that landed mercenaries in Black Beach Prison. The British National Archives in London had declassified their documents of "the *Albatross* affair." The archives were published for the first time in Adam Roberts's book, and evidence was extensive. It included a January 3, 1973, report out of Gibraltar alerting Britain to the plot. And documents found on board the *Albatross*. (Yes, the *Albatross*. Forsyth had even used that ship's name as one of those considered by the mercenaries in his novel.) Among other evidence, records of Forsyth's payments of large sums of money were found on board. Statements from men arrested showed that their plan matched the novel in every particular.

Over the years Forsyth has issued denial, followed by adjusted denial, followed by further adjusted denial. Confronted with evidence of his payments of large sums of money, he has claimed they were for information only. After Adam Roberts had gathered all his evidence, during his third interview with the novelist he bluntly asked Forsyth whether he plotted a coup in Equatorial Guinea. Roberts recounts that Forsyth laughed and said, "You put in the book what you have found."

It would seem the coup's success may be the only fiction in the novelists gripping tale. In real life the plot was foiled when authorities in the Canaries boarded the *Albatross*.

But *why*? If in fact he was involved, what motivated Forsyth? Carl and I and our friends favored the theory he wanted to create a home for the Igbo. Forsyth had reported from inside Biafra, so near Fernando Po, during their war of secession, and he became not just a reporter but a champion of the Biafra cause. So much so that he and the BBC had a parting of ways. Adding fuel to Forsyth's emotional fire, Equatorial Guinea had halted those Red Cross relief flights from Fernando Po, causing even greater suffering and starvation inside Biafra. That had been the very issue that precipitated the posting of Chargé d'Affaires Al Williams to Equatorial Guinea.

When Forsyth and a friend implicated in the coup attempt were tossing around the "what if" of the plan, Equatorial Guinea had become a more and more unbearable place to live. Conditions seemed right for a coup's success. Macias was feared and despised by his own people and hated by foreigners, all of whom would welcome his overthrow. The Igbo contract laborers, already the largest population group on Fernando Po, would applaud the brutal president's removal.

In 2015 Forsyth published his memoir, *The Outsider: My Life in Intrigue*. The book is a series of vivid stories of his work for MI6, Britain's equivalent of the CIA. In the chapter titled "Dogs of War," he says there was no need to "risk" going to Equatorial Guinea to research the novel because many who had been there gleefully shared information. Forsyth makes no reference to the claims he planned and financed an actual coup attempt. But the dust jacket's front flap entices the reader with the statement, "[Forsyth] was accused of helping to fund a coup in Equatorial Guinea."

Historian Randall Fegley ponders the larger picture in his authoritative book, *Equatorial Guinea: An African Tragedy*:

One cannot help but to think that the novelist and his

mercenary band had more insight than many in official positions. The fantastic dream of a new Biafra may have been unattainable . . . but both Forsyth and [the mercenary] knew the sort of government they were planning to destroy. While honorable statesmen and reputable businessmen were sweeping dirt under rugs, the vilified "dogs of war" attempted to end Equatorial Guinea's night of terror. (Fegley, p. 146)

Sadly, Macias Nguema would brutalize his people for eight more years after our departure. In 1979 he was executed after a bloody coup led by his nephew and right-hand man, Teodoro Obiang Nguema Mbasogo, who had personally supervised the administration of his uncle's atrocities and was a former governor of Black Beach Prison. He "returned the country to democracy," he said. But he has ruled ever since, always reelected by well over 90 percent of the vote.

Carl and I often talked about *The Dogs of War* and whether life would have been different for Equatorial Guineans had the coup succeeded.

Is life much better after the one that did?

———➤

A chronology of Macias's actions after we left can be found at the end of this book.

# 19

# HOME FROM THE FIELD

*He looked gaunt,* this man walking toward me from the plane. Clothes hung loose on his medium frame, and his sunken, olive-complexioned cheeks were red and wrinkled. A short, dark beard contrasted with thin sun-bleached hair. I took a closer look. The gait and tilt of the head were familiar, if not the beard and ill-fitting clothes. I squinted into the noonday glare to be sure this was my husband.

Carl had lost thirty pounds during his three months in Bangladesh. Our children and I, alone during this time, impatiently watched his approach. His slow pace conveyed exhaustion. But as he came close, I saw something else—a look of deep satisfaction. A glow.

In the coming days, that summer of 1975, as he talked about it in fragments, he would tell me of people dropping around him as he walked along a roadway. One dropping dead over here, one over there. Through the years, Carl had seen and heard and done things in healthcare that had etched images so deep they would never leave him—and now, Bangladesh.

He talked of inspecting every crumpled blanket along a road or a railway platform, looking for smallpox victims, alive or dead.

Piles of bodies, their ragged clothing their shrouds, were stacked like so many logs. Bodies awaiting someone. Or no one.

But the glow continued. Despite the horrors, Carl knew he had changed the fate of thousands. And thousands. He had seen some of the planet's last cases of variola major. And he had with him simple expressions of gratitude from the most vulnerable people on earth.

He had recorded on his Dictaphone, above the noise of his jeep traveling over rutted tracks, accounts of putting his bedroll on a table in a roadside guesthouse, the table legs sitting in something to repel rats. Or of sharing a tent with a Russian colleague as dedicated and passionate men and women on opposite sides of global conflict fought shoulder to shoulder in the cause to annihilate smallpox.

Sometimes, just when case numbers had plunged in Bangladesh and the finish line was in sight, the government would bulldoze acres of cardboard slums, or the lowlands would flood. Either event would send thousands on foot or riding on the tops of trains to anywhere-but-here, taking the virus to new groups of vulnerable people.

Carl kept going by telling himself what he had to do and never losing sight of the objective. A colleague in Bangladesh shared a journal entry about serving when all seems hopeless: "Dry-eyed compassion; tears diminish clarity of vision."

The haunting memories of Bangladesh might never leave him, and I believe he sometimes had to sit alone and cry. But neither would the sense of fulfillment leave him. In the foothills of the Himalayas, in steamy rain forest and in Sahel and savanna, he had given his all.

Our children and I had waited at home in Arizona while Carl worked in Bangladesh. Charles feared his dad wouldn't come back alive, and he often cried himself to sleep. Ginger remembers feeling sad for her dad's living conditions, especially his having to sleep on a table to avoid the rats, and worrying about the people of Bangladesh and what they must have to endure.

Just a few months after Carl returned home, on a remote Bangladesh island three-year-old Rahima Banu was diagnosed with killer smallpox. She survived what would turn out to be the world's last naturally occurring case of *variola major*. Two years later, in October 1977, a young hospital cook in Somalia, Ali Maow Maalin, survived the last naturally occurring case of *variola minor*. The long chain of smallpox transmission, dating back hundreds—if not thousands—of years, was ended.

After two more years of combing the planet to be sure no remaining virus lurked in some remote spot, the World Health Organization certified the world smallpox free. Global eradication of smallpox has been referred to as the equivalent of a "medical moonshot" and as "the single greatest achievement in the history of public health."

Cold War enemies had cooperated, or at least had worked out ways to function together to get the job done. In one example of Cold War tensions, Russians resented the American colleagues acting as though they had led the war on smallpox, and were quick to remind them that it was, in fact, the Soviets who had initially proposed global eradication of smallpox—back in 1958.

The triumph required medical science, obviously. It took masterful planning and administration. It took the physical and emotional sacrifices of an army of workers like Carl. And, yes, it took the price paid by their families to prevail against the killer.

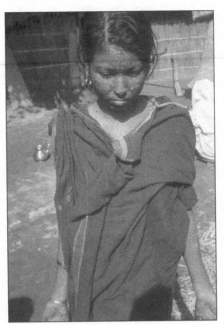

One of the world's last smallpox
victims, Bangladesh, 1975

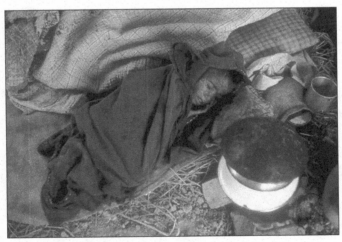

Smallpox victim lying beside the railroad track,
Bangladesh 1975

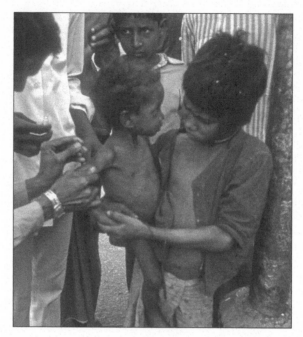

Vaccinating with the bifurcated needle

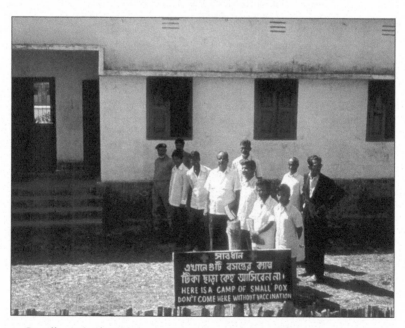

Smallpox isolation hospital Carl set up in Bangladesh, 1975

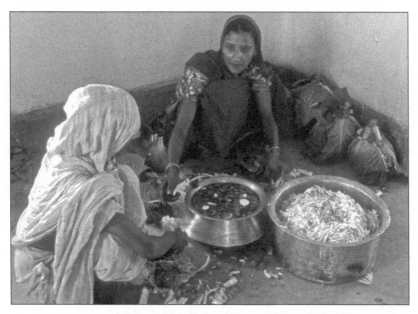

Families prepare food to be carried inside the hospital
by someone who is immune

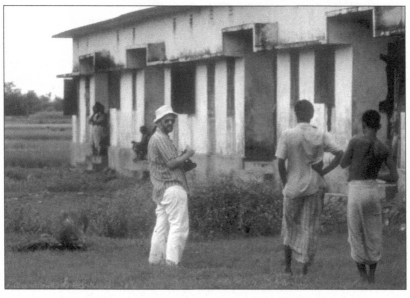

Carl visits the now boarded-up hospital after
global eradication, 1980

"*At a time of pessimism and unease, when the very notion of medical progress is being increasingly questioned, it is heartening to know that we stand poised for a triumph as great as any in the entire history of medicine: the total global eradication of smallpox*".  British Journal of Hospital Medicine, September 1975.

*The triumph belongs to an exceptional group of national workers and to a dedicated international staff from countries around the world who have shared privations and problems in pursuit of the common goal*

**SMALLPOX TARGET ZERO**

To *Carl H. Bloeser*

*one of the international staff who assisted the World Health Organization in this historic venture — the ORDER OF THE BIFURCATED NEEDLE is given as recognition of participation in this great achievement.*

*Geneva, 1976*

WHO Certificate celebrating the victory

# Reflection

Slide Show

As the projector hums I stare
at images on a cold, flat wall,

And I see images of human spirits
shattered by disease, and of
ambitions never found among eternal rice paddies,
For they have drowned in oppression of
a rainy season that never ends.

                     Carl Bloeser
                     (undated)

# 20

# THE FINAL CHAPTER

*2013*

"Where's that letter from Al?"

Carl is awake again. I squeeze his hand, stretch and get up from the napping chair I have placed against his bed.

"It's right here, honey," I say. "Here. Can you see it? In the black frame. Shall I read it to you again?"

No answer. He continues to search the many frames on the walls, his gaze less focused now as the brain cancer advances. Glioblastoma, the doctor said. Right frontal lobe. I said it was the last thing I wanted to hear. I know too much. Over the decades of my career I've treated too many patients with head injuries, cancers, strokes of the right frontal lobe. I know the road we will travel. And glioblastoma moves fast. We're saying good-bye.

His doctors tell us Carl's risk of falling is too great for him to be at home. We have no choice. The State Veteran Home allows us to personalize the rooms, so I've covered the walls with our life's history—photos, certificates, letters. Two walls are devoted to our family and our unique experiences. The other walls are testament to Carl's work in Nigeria, Equatorial Guinea, Bangladesh, the Indian Health Service, Saudi Arabia, Warsaw. Carl's career has taken him to or through more than seventy countries. I want to keep him anchored and reminded of what he's done and of the world he's shown us. I want him to remember he made a difference. Friends come and share fond memories that keep him reminded too.

"Are you thirsty? They just brought fresh water."

"—picture of the kids feeding the pigeons?"

"It's here. Under the little Christmas tree."

His eyes close. "I love that picture," he whispers, eyes still closed. "Is Charles here?"

"Not yet, honey. He'll be here this afternoon."

I search for a CD of Christmas carols. Carl wants to give a Christmas gift every time a caregiver comes into his room, so he gives them a CD and they slip it back in his drawer. Then the cycle is repeated.

"Where's that letter from Al?"

"It's right here," I say again.

He looks around.

I read to him once more a few lines from Al's two-page letter to CDC.

"[Carl's] success in dealing with two successive Ministers of Health, the latter of whom is known to be unfriendly to the West, singles out Mr. Bloeser—."

"—letter from the Indian Health Service?"

I read from that too. "Are you in pain, honey?"

He's moaning.

"This cool cloth will feel good on your face."

I adjust his quilt, a lovingly made gift from our church family that they've all signed. They have come often for comfort, times of worship and just their quiet presence. I settle back into my napping chair. I'm thankful to have this place to rest during the long days. Once nursing has settled Carl in for the night, I'll go home to sleep and come back in the morning.

As my attention drifts around the room, I ponder the mine-field of growing-up lessons Africa had waiting for me. Some that shook my foundations. I can hardly believe we lived that experience, and yet, here is photographic and documentary proof. Here are reminders of the fifty-three-year journey with my larger-than-life husband. I've had a comet by the tail, breathlessly holding on. My cutout-paper-doll notions of the world have given way to a three-dimensional tapestry full of color.

And even my former straightforward triumphalist narrative of eradicating smallpox is nuanced now. More complex. Indeed it was a triumph like none other. A global assault that defeated a killer virus. But with the lenses of hindsight and a wider perspective, I recognize that whereas smallpox and other diseases have often influenced power and politics, world powers use disease *fighters* to do the same.

Over the next few weeks, Carl detaches from his accomplishments. His few words are about me (he thinks I'm wonderful and tells everyone so) and about our children. Long ago he had to accept that neither wanted to be a doctor. But he was gratified that the life he had chosen to lead, and the example and experiences he had given our family, had instilled in both our children hearts of compassion and hands that acted on that compassion.

He's muttering something. I bend close.

"—hymns . . . play hymns."

I put on a CD. He's mouthing some of the words. And he likes me to read the Twenty-Third Psalm aloud—"The Lord is my shepherd. I shall not want . . ."—and his other favorite Bible passage, from the book of Romans:

> For I am convinced that neither death nor life, neither
> angels nor demons, neither the present nor the future, nor
> any powers, neither height nor depth, nor anything else

in all creation, will be able to separate us from the love
of God that is in Christ Jesus our Lord. (Romans 8:38–39,
NIV)

He's praying. His barely audible words are separated by si-
lences so long I keep thinking he's finished.

Charles and Ginger have come often since Carl's diagnosis,
and they reminisce with him about the lands and cultures we've
seen and the things we've done together. "Remember, Dad . . . ?
Remember the time we . . . ?"

Charles often sits with him for long hours and reads to him.

Ginger reminds him there's so much more to life than this life
and assures him we'll be together again. A moment of clarity returns to his eyes as he says, "I know."

Now both the kids and their families will gather here for
Christmas.

"—kids? Ginger coming?"

"Uh-huh. Everyone will be here, and we'll have dinner in
there by the big Christmas tree."

"—Courtney?"

He wants to see our granddaughter. "Sure. And I bet she'll
bring ice cream for her traditional treat with Grandpa."

Carl's dearly loved brother, Ken, travels across the country
again to see him. Carl has a spike in energy for Ken's visit. It lasts
for only a day.

His eyes seldom open now. It's different from when he left for
some far corner of the world. So many times I've seen this man
off. So many times I've said good-bye. I've become very independent through the years, and that will help. As I prepare to see him
off now, I'm secure in the confidence I'll see him again.

I'm rubbing his feet and looking around the room.

In a frame next to the photo of the now-boarded-up smallpox
isolation hospital Carl had set up in Bangladesh hangs my most

prized physical possession. It is a handwritten note on a yellowing piece of paper.

> FARE WEL TO. MR. BLOSER, RENOUNED PHELONTHROPIS
> WHO HAS COME OVER BANGLADESH TO HELP THE SEAK AND
> DISTRESS INDIVEDUALS WHO ARE AT THE ELEVENTH HOUR
> DUE TO POX DIESEASES.
>
> D. SIR,
>
> COMING FROM OVER SEAS TO HELP THE HELPLESS AND
> DISTRESS PEOPLE. YOU HAVE MADE AND ADVENTURE TO
> ERADICATE THIS DIESEASES FROM THIS COUNTRY. WE WILL
> NEVER FORGET YOU AND YOUR ART OF TREATMENT TO US.
> LONG LEAVE YOU. WISH YOUR BETTER PROSPECT LATER LIFE
>
> THANK YOU.
>
> DATED MYM.
> THE 22ND MARCH, 75.
>
> AFFECTIONATELY YOUR'S
> THE WORKERS. OF THE LOCAL HEALTH
> ORGANIZATION SPONCHORED BY W.H-O
> OVER MYMENSINGH.

The speech pathologist had worked with Carl when there was hope of reaching any functional goal. Since therapy has ended, she continues to drop by for a few minutes after her workday. Today when Carl doesn't open his eyes or speak, she focuses on his face and the information his features communicate. When his brow is furrowed, she starts through a list:

"Ginger is okay. Charles is okay. Bee has the finances in order," she says. When she still sees worry in his face, she continues, "Bee is okay, and we're sending her home. We're making sure she gets enough rest." Only then do his muscles relax.

She tells me Carl is still trying to take care of me.

I settle into my chair and lock my fingers with his.

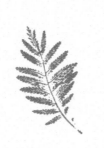

# EPILOGUE

## On Writing *Vaccines & Bayonets*

*The church was* filled that day. People had come to celebrate the life of my husband. Our minister read the biographical summary I had written, and after the service several people asked for a copy. They'd had no idea what Carl had done in his life. I asked them to wait until I could write something a little more complete. About ten pages should do it, I thought.

It was a few months before I could face going through Carl's filing cabinets. When I finally got to the drawer of carefully preserved archives from our years in West Africa, I read through hundreds of pages, every shred. That's when I knew—I had to write the book.

He was always going to write it, you see. The book. But cancer aborted his dreams and took his life. So there I sat, four months after Carl's passing, staring into the black screen of an iPad. The one the hospital therapist recommended for Carl's cognitive exercises. But brain cancer had raced ahead—too fast. My book is different than his would have been, but I was determined to pick up the baton.

When I set out to tell our family's Africa story, I didn't anticipate the emotional and physical reactions I would have reliving the sight of the mass grave in Kano and our stress and isolation in Equatorial Guinea. In addition, sleepy little Santa Isabel was far more tragic than I even knew, the depth and intensity of its suffering hidden from me. Reading descriptions of the tortures and the methods of execution being practiced half a mile from our house made me literally ill, and I have had sleepless nights when those details refused to stay in my filing cabinets as mere words on sheets of paper.

The stories in this memoir take place at the intersection of people, places and programs. With the exception of background characters, none are composites. To protect their identities, I changed the names of Equatorial Guineans who worked for the Americans. I used place names that were current during our time in West Africa. No attempt has been made to give a complete chronicle of every person encountered or every event.

In supplementing my own archives through external research on Equatorial Guinea, contradictory information among sources was a frustration. Furthermore, in those sources, no matter how well researched and documented, I found some statements that I know to be in error because I experienced the event firsthand. But contradictions are doubtless unavoidable among writers, no matter how scholarly the attempts. I have done my best to follow the trail of references to find the most authoritative document. In some cases, that trail ended in my filing cabinets.

There are several possible reasons for contradictions in addition to the fact that any two people reporting on the same event may differ in the way they perceive and remember that event.

First, many of the primary sources available are in Spanish and there may be errors in translation. Second, it is recognized that official primary source documents are sometimes not true to the facts because of political motivations.

Third, a cloak of secrecy descended on Equatorial Guinea beginning within six months of the country's independence. In March 1969, President Macias shut down presses, imposed severe censorship and banned all foreign journalists from entering the country. Other travelers could rarely obtain visas. In January 1971, Francoist Spain "classified" all news and comment about Equatorial Guinea. Any mention of their former colony in the press was in violation of Spain's Official Secrets Act. Because of this secrecy and people's fear to speak out, many writings are based at least in part on a third party's written or verbal report, some of which have limited possibility of confirmation.

In the case of my own book, I have written my personal perceptions of events I witnessed, information told to us when we were there and information we wrote into our notes as events or conversations occurred. Those reports were close to the source in time and place. That does not make them, or our hearing of them, infallible.

Working with the above challenges, I have made every effort to tell as accurate a story as I believe possible.

## The Biological Warfare and Climate Change Concerns

Smallpox, the disease, is gone. The *variola* virus still exists. Tragically, the last death from smallpox occurred a year after the last naturally occurring case. In a medical school in Birmingham, England, the virus escaped a laboratory, through the ventilation system it is believed. It infected medical photographer, Janet Parker, working one floor below. Subsequently, all laboratories were instructed to send any remaining samples of the virus to a central repository.

The legal vials are in freezers in only two highly secure

laboratories, one in the United States and one in Russia. Since WHO declared the world smallpox free in 1980, a debate has raged about which better protects us—completely destroying the virus or keeping the samples for research? To the date of this writing, the latter view has prevailed.

The US government stages exercises like "Dark Winter" to try to gauge our preparedness should the virus escape the laboratory, accidentally or otherwise, into a world population that is no longer immune. And these exercises assess our preparedness for other pandemics.

We know that scientific tools of "dark biology" grow ever more sophisticated. We know that the DNA of variola and other deadly viruses can be weaponized, made more lethal. Synthetic biology may have been the stuff of science fiction a few years ago. It's no longer fiction.

Bill Gates speaks of epidemic preparedness at the World Economic Forum, Davos. Preparedness for pandemics—like COVID-19 and those we can't yet conceive of.

And now, with some of the world's previously frozen areas beginning to thaw, scientists look at the possibility of reintroduction of old diseases, including release of the smallpox virus.

We should pray that the demon stays locked in the freezer, and in the tundra, and that the world never again sees the speckled monster.

## So What Happened to the Dictator?

Historians have asserted that Macias was worse than Idi Amin or Pol Pot in the extent of his atrocities, and that he killed proportionately more people than did Hitler. Amnesty International workers began to nickname Equatorial Guinea the Auschwitz of Africa and the Dachau of Africa. Gathered from historians, here is a sampling of Macias's actions after our family left Equatorial Guinea.

| | |
|---|---|
| **February 1972** | Presidential portrait was found slashed at a Bata school and anti-Macias slogans on blackboards in others, so Macias executed the new minister of education in the streets of Santa Isabel and publicly displayed his body. |
| **May 1972** | Purge continued. Macias imprisoned ministry of health's technical director and chief auditor of the Central Bank; auditor was later decapitated. |
| **July 14, 1972** | Macias staged a sham election, made himself president-for-life. |
| **March 1973** | Macias allowed half the population of tiny, remote Annobón to die in cholera epidemic before he agreed to send vaccine. |
| **July 1973** | Third National Congress of the One Political Party approved new constitution. Macias was granted the power to veto all legislation, to declare war, to appoint and dismiss all judges, civil servants, diplomats and military officers. Repealed all constitutional safeguards protecting the island minorities. Voting day to approve this was "indescribable terror." Anyone intending to abstain or vote against was threatened with public killing. The few who abstained were beaten, and survivors were executed a few days later. Macias then had absolute personal power. |

**Other in 1973**    Macias had the island of Fernando Po named after him, Macias Nguema Biyogo. He controlled the radio and press, prohibited foreign travel. Accused United Nations Development Programme (UNDP) of plotting against his government, ordered them shut down after finding "suspicious documents." The UNDP director and his staff were beaten when he refused to turn over UN papers; their chauffeur was killed.

**June 13, 1974**    Alleged a coup attempt in Bata Jail; killed 118 prisoners and many others. After one visit to Bata Jail, Macias said the prisoners were being "spoiled" and they should not be "treated so well." (Date unknown.)

**Nov, 1974**    Macias banned all public religious meetings. Clergy who hadn't fled were imprisoned; some church buildings became cacao sheds. Cathedral became an arsenal.

**Feb. 12, 1975**    Macias's picture above the vice president's office was found torn; he ordered the VP publicly tortured and shot.

**March 18, 1975**    Banned private education.

**1975**    In speech in Bata, Macias said women were not to talk politics.

Juventud whipped entire Nigerian embassy staff; militia killed eleven Nigerians in their own embassy's garden. Nigeria repatriated its nationals by plane and by ship; soldiers opened fire on them in the harbor.

**Christmas 1975**    Macias once again used the stadium to execute "subversives." Executioners in Santa Claus costumes killed at least 150, again to the strains of "Those Were the Days."

**1975–77**    Increase in arrests and summary executions.
Arrests for "failing to attend national manifestations of praise and joy."

| | |
|---|---|
| **July 7, 1976** | Macias publicly executed governor of Central Bank; closed Central Bank. Took national treasure to his home in rural Rio Muni. Paid government employees out of his suitcases, if at all. |
| **Unknown date** | By the time the last schools were closed, Macias had expelled all teachers and replaced them with loyal clan members; only subject taught was "Adoration of Macias." |
| **1978** | Changed the country's motto to "There is no other God than Macias Nguema." |
| | Instituted capital punishment for any attempt to attack the president, thirty years' imprisonment for accomplices, and punishment for insulting or offending the president. |
| **June 1979** | A group of five Guardia Nacional came to Macias to petition for their eight months' backlog of pay. Macias had them executed. |
| **August 3, 1979** | Lt. Col. Teodoro Obiang Nguema Mbasogo, who was Macias's right-hand man, vice minister of defense and military governor of Bioko Province, ousted his uncle, Macias Nguema, in a bloody coup. Macias was cornered in his hideout in rural Rio Muni with what was left of the national treasury. He escaped into the rain forest. (Some sources, but not all, assert he set the hut ablaze as soldiers closed in, burning the cash remaining in the treasury.) His wife, as she had done at times in the past, crossed the border with several suitcases full of money. |
| | While the junta soldiers searched the forest for Macias, Obiang announced the coup. People danced in the long-deserted streets; jubilant crowds at the airport shook the hands of journalists arriving to cover the coup. Churches were reopened and hundreds stood in line to have their children baptized. |

**August 18, 1979**   Soldiers captured Macias near the Gabonese border, imprisoned him in Bata, then transferred him to Black Beach Prison.

**Sept. 24, 1979**   Trial began in Santa Isabel (named Malabo by that time).

Historian Randall Fegley reports that by the end of Macias's rule, 110,000 people (total reported population when we arrived was 260,000) had gone into exile, and his regime had murdered 20,000 people at the very least. Included in that number were:

- eighteen cabinet ministers
- twenty-two members of national and provincial assemblies
- seven mayors and local councilors
- five ambassadors
- seventy-five teachers and school administrators
- forty of the forty-six members of the 1967 Constitutional Conference
- spouses and other relatives of all of the above

More than two thirds of the first legislative assembly died violently or disappeared.

Twelve or more villages suffered mass executions and had been burned or pillaged.

Further detail is presented by these authors listed in the Sources Consulted:

Artuccio, Alejandro
Cronje, Suzanne
Fegley, Randall
Klinteberg, Robert af
Liniger-Goumaz, Max

Detail about the tortures and executions are given by these authors in Sources Consulted:

Brabazon, James
Fegley, Randall
Roberts, Adam

## Trial of Macias

The military tribunal of Macias and ten accomplices lasted for five days. Obiang, the leader of the coup and president of the Supreme Military Council, in a veneer of openness, invited the International Commission of Jurists (ICJ) to send an observer to the trial. ICJ designated Dr. Alejandro Artuccio of Uruguay for that task and published his detailed account of the conditions he found in the country, along with details and analysis of the trial itself.

When Dr. Artuccio arrived in Equatorial Guinea, he found a paralyzed country: no power lines, phones or other public services. Ninety percent of public administration was no longer functioning. Public officials' meager salaries were paid eight or nine months late. Officials, like everyone else, had to search for food in the forest. Public offices, buildings for schools, hospitals and offices were all idle or abandoned. He found not a single restaurant and only empty shelves in the few remaining stores (State trading posts).

Over the course of the trial, the Supreme Military Counsel gradually reduced its charges as the accused tried to spread the blame, pointing fingers back at the accusers. Dr. Artuccio states the "most salient defect" of the trial was that only a few of the guilty were brought before the tribunal. Historian Dr. Arnold Fegley states accusations covered only the period 1969 to 1974.

After that date, most of the members of the junta were involved in the terror.

The reader wanting more detail about the trial of Macias may wish to go to these authors listed in Sources Consulted:

Artuccio, Alejandro

Fegley, Randall

## After the Trial

Besides those who crowded into the theater where the trial took place, thousands followed the proceedings through loudspeakers in the streets. They initially celebrated when they heard the conviction and pronouncement of sentence, but their joy soon mingled with fear. Macias had convinced people he had a powerful spirit and would come back to haunt them if he was killed. Locals were afraid to carry out the death penalty. Moroccan soldiers were hired as the firing squad.

The new government, headed by Macias's nephew, Lieutenant Colonel Teodoro Obiang Nguema Mbasogo, who had personally supervised administration of Macias-ordered torture and executions, said they had released all political prisoners immediately after the coup. But the number of those released was in dispute, with Amnesty International maintaining that a large number were summarily executed rather than released.

President Obiang said he would return the country to democracy "as soon as possible," but "until the economy was working again no political activity could be tolerated." He said all of the exiled Guineans (approximately 110,000) were welcome to return, but that they had to accept those conditions. Few of the exiled trusted him or accepted his offer.

## And Then There Was Oil

In 1995 the discovery of prodigious oil reserves sitting under the tiny country propelled Equatorial Guinea into the spotlight of the world's petro-drama. It is one of the largest oil producers in Africa and has one of the highest GDPs.

Obiang has ruled for more than forty years. He is repeatedly accused of corruption, election fraud and brutal oppression of opposition voices. His son, Teodoro Obiang Nguema Mangue (nickname Teodorín), is vice president, heir apparent and international playboy. He is known for his ostentatious lifestyle, spending his country's oil wealth on 250-foot yachts, fleets of luxury cars, and mansions in the world's most exclusive enclaves.

Half or more of the country's population lives in poverty and has no electricity or safe drinking water. Multiple sources report 40 percent of children are not in school.

The reader interested in the history of Equatorial Guinea during and since the rule of Macias is encouraged to read further from Other Sources Consulted and Suggested Readings.

# ACRONYMS AND ABBREVIATIONS

**CDC**    Centers for Disease Control and Prevention (1992) (see NCDC)

**DCM**    deputy chief of mission

**EG**    Equatorial Guinea

**FSO**    foreign service officer

**GOEG**    government of Equatorial Guinea

**NCDC**    National Communicable Disease Center (changed to Centers for Disease Control in 1970)

**OAU**    Organization of African Unity

**OCEAC**    Organization of Coordination for the Fight Against Endemic Diseases in Central Africa

**SEP**    Smallpox Eradication Program

**SMP**    Smallpox/Measles Program

**UNDP**    United Nations Development Programme

**USAID**    United States Agency for International Development

**WHA**    World Health Assembly

**WHO**    World Health Organization

# SOURCES

## Unclassified primary documents in the author's personal archives

- Personal diary/journal notes, letters to family, and newsletters to family and friends
- Collected cables and letters exchanged between Carl Bloeser and Ambassador Hoffacker, Chargé d'Affaires Al Williams, USAID, and CDC
- Collected cables and letters exchanged between Ambassador Hoffacker and USAID
- Collected reports and letters from Chargé d'Affaires Al Williams
- Monthly Activity Reports from Carl Bloeser to CDC and to the government of Equatorial Guinea
- Equatorial Guinea End of Tour Report from Carl Bloeser to CDC
- Letter from Chargé d'Affaires Williams to Dr. David Sencer, director of CDC
- CDC response to Chargé d'Affaires Williams from Dr. Bill Foege

- Smallpox/measles program proposal: Carl Bloeser to the government of Equatorial Guinea
- Text of speech by President Macias on anniversary of independence (English translation from the Fang)
- Text of speech by President Macias on anniversary of the Single National Party (PUN) (English translation from the Fang)
- Incident report from Wolfgang Schorcht to UNDP
- Collected notes and invitations from embassies in Equatorial Guinea
- Letter from Jean Roy to CDC
- Letter from Chargé d'Affaires Alfred Erdos to the government of Equatorial Guinea
- Letter from Rosita Leahy
- Author's handwritten notes made during telephone call from Rosita Leahy
- Author's handwritten notes made during telephone call from Jean Erdos
- Assorted State Department articles and newspaper articles
- Cassette tape letters to family
- Email from Al Williams to the author
- Film of Carl Bloeser and his teams working in northern Nigeria
- Bloeser, Carl. "A Review of the West and Central African Smallpox Eradication Measles Control Program." Master's thesis, University of Texas, 1973.

## Interviews

- In-person interviews with Dr. Joyce Bradley: 2014–2018
- In-person interviews with Al Williams: Oct. 19, 2014, Oct. 23–24, 2015

- Telephone interview with Al Williams: Aug. 18, 2016
- Email correspondence with Carman (Williams) Cunning-ham: September 2016

# OTHER SOURCES CONSULTED / SUGGESTED READING

## Smallpox and smallpox eradication sources

Bowen, Elenore Smith (Laura Bohanan). *Return to Laughter: An Anthropological Novel.* New York: Anchor Books, 1964.

Brilliant, Larry. *Sometimes Brilliant: The Impossible Adventure of a Spiritual Seeker and Visionary Physician Who Helped Conquer the Worst Disease in History.* New York: HarperCollins, 2016.

Carrell, Jennifer Lee. *The Speckled Monster: A Historical Tale of Battling Smallpox.* New York: Penguin, 2004.

Foege, William H. *House on Fire: The Fight to Eradicate Smallpox.* Berkeley: University of California Press, 2011.

Henderson, D. A. *Smallpox—The Death of a Disease: The Inside Story of Eradicating a Worldwide Killer.* New York: Prometheus Books, 2009.

Joarder, A. K., D. Tarantola, and J. Tulloch. "The Eradication of Smallpox from Bangladesh." New Delhi: World Health Organization, South-East Asia Regional Office, 1980.

Ogden, Horace G. "CDC and the Smallpox Crusade." Washington, DC: US Department of Health and Human Services, 1987.

Preston, Richard. *The Demon in the Freezer: A True Story*. New York: Random House, 2003.

Reinhardt, Bob H. *The End of a Global Pox: America and the Eradication of Smallpox in the Cold War Era*. Durham: University of North Carolina Press, 2015.

## Nigeria

Adichie, Chimamanda Ngozi. *Half of a Yellow Sun*. New York: Alfred A. Knopf-Random House, 2006.

Forsyth, Frederick. *The Making of an African Legend: The Biafra Story*. London: Penguin, 1969.

Kencke, J., and Sally Hesling (index and foreword). *Crocodile: Recipes from the International Women's Club, Kaduna, Nigeria, Africa*. 1981.

Madauci, Ibrahim, Yahaya Isa, and Bello Daura. *Hausa Customs*. Zaria: Northern Nigeria Publishing, 1968.

Ministry of Information, Kano State. *Kano State of Nigeria*. Kano, 1969.

Orr, Elaine Neil. *Gods of Noonday: A White Girl's African Life*. Charlottesville: University of Virginia Press, 2003.

## Equatorial Guinea

Amnesty International. All reports on Equatorial Guinea.

Artucio, Dr. Alejandro. *The Trial of Macias in Equatorial Guinea: The Story of a Dictatorship*. The International Commission of Jurists, International University Exchange Fund, 1979.

Brabazon, James. *My Friend the Mercenary: A Memoir*. New York: Grove Press, 2011.

Burton, Sir Richard Francis. *Wanderings in West Africa, from Liverpool to Fernando Po*. Cambridge: Cambridge University Press, 2011.

London: Tinsley, 1863. Reissue edition: New York: Dover Publications, 1991.

Cronje, Suzanne. *Equatorial Guinea: The Forgotten Dictatorship.* London: Anti-Slavery Society, 1976.

Fegley, Randall. *Equatorial Guinea: An African Tragedy.* New York: Peter Lang Publishing, 1989.

———. *International Action against Genocide*, Report #53. London: Minority Rights Group, 1984.

———. "Minority Oppression in Equatorial Guinea." In *World Minorities Vol. II.* London: Minority Rights Group, 1978.

———. "The UN Human Rights Commission: The Equatorial Guinea Case." *The Human Rights Quarterly* 3, (Fall 1981): 81–100.

Forsyth, Frederick. *The Dogs of War.* New York: Viking Press, 1974.

———. *The Outsider: My Life in Intrigue.* New York: Putnam, 2015.

Garthoff, Raymond L. *A Journey through the Cold War: A Memoir of Containment and Coexistence.* Washington, DC: Brookings Institution Press, 2001.

Hochschild, Adam. *Bury the Chains: The British Struggle to Abolish Slavery.* London: Macmillan, 2005.

Hoyt, Michael P. E. *Captive in the Congo: A Consul's Return to the Heart of Darkness.* Annapolis, MD: Naval Institute Press, 2000.

Kingsley, Mary. *Travels in West Africa.* New York: Macmillan, 1897.

Klinteberg, Robert af. *Equatorial Guinea-Macias Country: The Forgotten Refugees.* Geneva: International University Exchange Fund, 1978.

Klitgaard, Robert. *Tropical Gangsters: One Man's Experience with Development and Decadence in Deepest Africa.* New York: Basic Books, 1990.

Liniger-Goumaz, Max. *Small Is Not Always Beautiful: The Story of*

*Equatorial Guinea.* Translated by John Wood. Washington, DC: Rowman & Littlefield, 1988.

Repinecz, Martin. "Labyrinths of memories: A conversation with Francisco Zamora Loboch." *The Postcolonialist,* June 25, 2014.

Roberts, Adam. *The Wonga Coup: Guns, Thugs and a Ruthless Determination to Create Mayhem in an Oil-Rich Corner of Africa.* New York: Public Affairs, 2006.

Sundiata, Ibrahim K. *From Slaving to Neo-Slavery: The Bight of Biafra and Fernando Po in the Era of Abolition, 1827–1930.* Madison: University of Wisconsin Press, 1996.

Ugarte, Michael. *Africans in Europe: The Culture of Exile & Emigration from Equatorial Guinea to Spain.* Chicago: University of Illinois Press, 2010.

## Other

Kennan, George F. "Diplomacy as a Profession." *Foreign Service Journal,* May 1961.

## Television productions

BBC. "The Frontline Club. Adam Roberts—the Wonga Coup." April 1, 2007. YouTube video. 1:05, https://www.youtube.com/watch?v=V8FnoUHfBUI

BBC News. "Frederick Forsyth. My Days as an MI6 Spy." August 30, 2015. YouTube video. 3:21, https://www.youtube.com/watch?v=LbsKGvUDlHs

CBS News. "60 Minutes. Issues Behind the Nigeria-Biafra War." June 10, 1969. YouTube video. 60, https://www.youtube.com/watch?v=O7ymYBuqac0&ab_channel=reelblack

## Internet sources

Association for Diplomatic Studies and Training (ADST). "Moments in Diplomatic History: Murder in an Embassy, Part

I—'I am not losing my mind.'" https://adst.org/2013/09/i-am-not-losing-my-mind-murder-in-an-embassy-part-i/

Association for Diplomatic Studies and Training (ADST). "Moments in Diplomatic History: Murder in an Embassy, Part II—Paranoid Psychotic or Faked Insanity?" https://adst.org/2013/09/murder-in-an-embassy-part-ii-paranoid-psychotic-or-faked-insanity/

Association for Diplomatic Studies and Training (ADST). "Oral History Interviews with: Ambassador Raymond L. Garthoff, John E. Graves, Ambassador Lewis Hoffacker, Michael P. E. Hoyt, Carroll Sherer (widow of Ambassador Albert W. "Bud" Sherer Jr.) and Ambassador Leonard Shurtleff." https://adst.org/oral-history/

Global Health Chronicles. "Oral History Interviews with: William Foege, Paula Foege, Stanley Foster, Billy Griggs, D. A. Henderson, Jim Hicks, Don Millar, Betty Roy, Jean Roy." https://globalhealthchronicles.org/smallpox-eradication

McKenna, Maryn. "Child Mummy Found with Oldest Known Smallpox Virus." *National Geographic.* https://www.nationalgeographic.com/news/2016/12/mummies-smallpox-virus-dna-lithuania-health-science/

# ACKNOWLEDGMENTS

*Many people have* given of their expertise, time, energy and friendship to help make this book a reality. I owe more than I can express, but I make the attempt.

My very talented granddaughter, Courtney Ann, contributed the book's outstanding front cover design.

My son, Charles, with his writing and editing skill helped me chart an early course. From the day he was reading my first attempts and I said, "This is when you're supposed to say, 'Wow, Mom!'" he gave me critique and perspective instead. I can't thank him enough.

My dear friend and mentor, Dr. Sandy Kaser, has been by my side from the beginning. I'm thankful she agreed to take me on. She taught, edited, prodded and encouraged. She provided writing retreats in the pines. Joe Sweeney and his writing group encouraged and coached, even before I had written a word.

Members of my critique groups, especially that intrepid group of nonfiction Rillito River Writers, helped me alter my decades-long clinical report style, reading and polishing chapter by chapter. I wish I could name each individual member.

My wonderful beta readers provided invaluable feedback: Stephanie Dorfman, Amy Fink, Janis Hunnicutt, Deb Liggett,

Fred Mezger, Dr. Martha Miller, Andrea Owan and Roy and Sandy Walkinshaw. A second group of readers reviewed the manuscript after I discovered new information that required additions to the text: Jeanne Dursi, my sister, Peggy Lee, Wendy Council, Mimi Villafane and Mary Lou Forier.

The volunteers at SCORE coached me in the business side of writing a book. Troy and DJ Berlin provided much-needed tech assistance. Mary Lou Forier and Tammy Bose exhibited infinite patience in formatting my manuscript for submission.

Pulitzer-nominated author, Pamela Alexander, reviewed and commented on the manuscript. And accepted yet another phone call to answer yet another question.

Andrea Owan and Elizabeth Leah Reed, friends and professional editors, gifted me with many hours of their time and expertise to ready the manuscript for submission, and Elizabeth did an edit of the full manuscript before my sending it to the publisher. My daughter, Ginger Elliott, lent her skills to rounds of edits with the publisher.

Ethel Lee-Miller reviewed the manuscript but also gave me the platform to present public readings of my book chapters at her Writers Read events. She and Sally Lanyon were by my side, nurturing and encouraging. Glenda Bonin and the others in Tucson Tellers of Tales provided a receptive audience and feedback for polishing the oral telling of many of these stories.

Pepperdine University Harbor Lectures, Santa Barbara Yacht Club Monday Forums, and various chapters of P.E.O., Toastmasters International, Sisters in Crime and Delta Kappa Gamma have been receptive audiences for my book-related lectures.

Through their own books, two historians and three of the heroes who led the smallpox fight fleshed out my background research, filled in gaps in my memory or confirmed sketchy information I had written in my letters and cryptic notes: Jennifer Lee Carrell in *The Speckled Monster*, Bob Reinhardt in *The End of a Global Pox*, Dr. D. A. Henderson in *Death of a Disease*, Dr. Bill Foege in *House on Fire*, and Dr. Larry Brilliant in *Sometimes Brilliant*. CDC's oral histories from these and other colleagues and spouses served to further jog my memory.

Among historians, Randall Fegley, in *Equatorial Guinea: An African Tragedy*, did the most to shine a light on the hidden atrocities that were unfolding around me, but of which I was blissfully ignorant at the time.

Adam Roberts, *Economist* Midwest Correspondent and author of *The Wonga Coup* and *Superfast Primetime Ultimate Nation*, shared with me some of his own research about Equatorial Guinea.

Sasha Polakow-Suransky, Deputy Editor of *Foreign Policy* magazine and author of *The Unspoken Alliance* and *Go Back to Where You Came From*, believed in my book and offered suggestions, encouragement and contacts.

Lara Weisweiller-Wu, editor for London's scholarly press, Hurst Publishing, devoted time to reading my manuscript and offered her validation and encouragement on my path to publication.

The Society of Southwestern Authors chose earlier versions of two memoir chapters as winners in their 2015 contest and included them in their anthology, *The Storyteller 2015: A Publication of the Society of Southwestern Authors*.

These individuals provided significant support to help get *Vaccines & Bayonets* published: Mary Lou Forier, Deb Liggett, Alex Alexander, Amy Fink, Peggy and David Lee, Peggy Huffman, Ginger and David Elliott, Ken Bloeser, Charles Bloeser, Sharon Anderson, Sandy Kaser, Andrea Owan, Nancy Jewett, Carol Teal, Claudia Lorber, Sally Krusing, Nelson and Julie Dorfman,

Gayland and Lis Yarbrough, Jeanne Porter, Angela and Bill El-liott, Rebecca and Russ Debenport, James and Julie Delcamp, the Curry and Barnard families, and Linda and Tom Hall.

Wheatmark Publishing, including Sam Henrie, Lori Conser and the rest of the team, brought their expertise and professionalism to my manuscript to put a polished product into your hands.

I extend profound thanks to dear friends who appear in this memoir and with whom I share a unique bond of life in a far-off time and place. During my writing of this book, we've shared conversations rich with memories: Al Williams, Carman (Williams) Cunningham and Dr. Joyce Bradley.

And finally, I thank family members and friends for tolerating me, supporting me and loving me over these years of writing. I so appreciate their avoiding, or at least hiding, the glazed-eye look when I managed to somehow turn yet another conversation in the direction of my book. Thank you one and all.

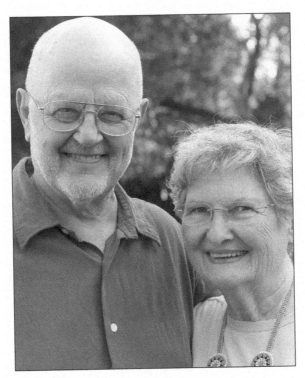

Carl and Bee, 2011

Made in USA - Kendallville, IN
95191_9781627878562
12.22.2022 1446